Narjes ABID
Sabrine BERRAZGA

Pleural tuberculosis: epidemiological, clinical and evolutionary aspects

Narjes ABID
Sabrine BERRAZGA

Pleural tuberculosis: epidemiological, clinical and evolutionary aspects

ScienciaScripts

Cover image: www.ingimage.com

This book is a translation from the original published under ISBN 978-620-6-72317-2.

Publisher:
Sciencia Scripts
is a trademark of
Dodo Books Indian Ocean Ltd. and OmniScriptum S.R.L publishing group

120 High Road, East Finchley, London, N2 9ED, United Kingdom
Str. Armeneasca 28/1, office 1, Chisinau MD-2012, Republic of Moldova, Europe
Managing Directors: Ieva Konstantinova, Victoria Ursu
info@omniscriptum.com

Printed at: see last page
ISBN: 978-620-8-52962-8

TABLE OF CONTENTS

LIST OF ABBREVIATIONS

TB: tuberculosis

HIV: human immunodeficiency virus **WHO:** World Health Organization **EPTB**: extra-pulmonary tuberculosis

LP: Pleural fluid

BCG: Bacille de Calmette et Guérin

IDR: Intradermal Reaction

CBC: blood count

R: Rifampicin

H: Isoniazid

Z: Pyrazinamide

E: Ethambutol

HTA: Hypertension

CT: computed tomography

BAAR: acid-fast bacilli

BP: Pleural biopsy

PNLT: National Tuberculosis Control Program

BTS: Britisc thoracic society

IFN: Interferon gamma

ADA 2: adenosine deaminase 2 isoenzyme

ADA: Total adenosine deaminase

PCR: polymerase chain reaction

IGRA: the interferon-gamma release

LDH: lactate dehydrogenase

IL-6: interleukin 6
IL-1α: interleukin 1 alpha

TNFα: tumor necrosis factor alpha

TOD: directly observed therapy

MDR-TB: multidrug-resistant tuberculosis

EFR: functional respiratory exploration

ADF: fixed drug association

INTRODUCTION

Tuberculosis (TB) continues to represent a major public health problem, both nationally and internationally, due to its high frequency on the one hand, and the significant morbidity and mortality it entails on the other. It is the 13th leading cause of death from all causes, and ranks second among infectious diseases worldwide, after COVID-19 and ahead of AIDS [1].

Pulmonary involvement remains by far the most common form of tuberculosis. However, there is currently a resurgence of extra-pulmonary involvement, particularly in regions human immunodeficiency virus (HIV) infection has become more common [2].

In 2020, the World Health Organization (WHO) reported 5.8 million new cases of tuberculosis, 18% of which were extra pulmonary [1].

Tunisia, a country with intermediate TB endemicity, has also seen an increase in the number of new cases of extra-pulmonary TB (EPTB) from 727 in 2000 to 2052 in 2017 [3]. In 2017, extra-pulmonary TB accounted for 62% of all forms of tuberculosis [4]

Pleural localization is among the most common extra-pulmonary localizations adults. In 2018, pleural TB accounted for 52% of all extra-pulmonary localizations [5]. However, this form of tuberculosis is little studied in the literature. Its diagnosis is often difficult due to its pauci-bacillary nature and the need, sometimes, for invasive procedures for biopsy samples. [6]

In the current context, where the incidence of pleural TB is on the rise in our country, knowledge of its different radio-clinical presentations, as well as its various diagnostic and therapeutic modalities, seems essential.

In this context we conducted a retrospective study of 50 cases of pleural TB collected at the Pneumology Department of CHU Mohamed Taher Maamouri Nabeul over a 4-year period from January 2015 to December 2019.

The objectives of our work were to describe the epidemiological profile of pleural TB in Cap Bon, to identify its clinical features and to specify its therapeutic and evolutionary modalities.

METHODS

1. Type and duration study :

We conducted a descriptive retrospective study of 50 records of patients with pleural TB that was diagnosed and followed at the Pneumology Department of CHU Mohamed Taher Maamouri Nabeul over a 4-year period from January 2015 until December 2019.

2. Inclusion criteria :

Patients presenting with isolated tuberculous pleurisy or pleurisy associated with parenchymal involvement, confirmed by anatomopathological study (tuberculoid granulomas with or without caseous necrosis) and/or bacteriological study (BAAR on direct examination and/or mycobacterium tuberculosis on pleural fluid (LP) culture) or molecular biology were included in the study.

3. Non-inclusion criteria :

Patients with pleurisy associated with pulmonary tuberculosis whose tuberculosis status has not been confirmed by bacteriological examination of the LP and/or pathological examination of the pleura.

Patients under 15 years of age (this age is not covered by
in our department).

4. Data collection :

Data were collected from patients' medical records. These data were transmitted on an analytical form containing the following headings:

1) Socio-demographic data: surname, first name, age, gender, origin, profession, educational level, socioeconomic level.

2) Personal and family history, as well as lifestyle habits (smoking, alcohol and other types of addiction, time spent in prison).

3) Bacille Calmette-Guérin (BCG) vaccination status.

4) Clinical data: time to consultation (time between onset of clinical signs and consultation), functional and general signs, physical signs.

5) The result of the tuberculin intradermal skin test (IDR). The IDR is considered positive if the diameter of the induration at the tuberculin injection site at 48-72h exceeds 10mm.

6) Results of para-clinical investigations: biological, radiological, bacteriological and

anatomopathological.

-LP features :

❖ Result of biochemical study specifying the level of protides in the LP. Exudative pleurisy is defined by a protide level in the LP greater than 35g/l or between 25 and 35g/l associated with one of the following criteria: Light's criteria [7].

- LP proteins divided by serum proteins> 0.5
- LP LDH divided by serum LDH> 0.6
- Pleural LDH levels above 200 IU/ml.

❖ Cytological findings: cellularity and cell count. Lymphocyte predominance is defined as a lymphocyte/white cell count in the LP > 50%.

❖ Results of bacteriological examination (direct examination - molecular biology PCR study - culture).

7) Biopsy technique used: surgical per thoracoscopy or percutaneous pleural biopsy with Abrams needle (figure 1) [8].

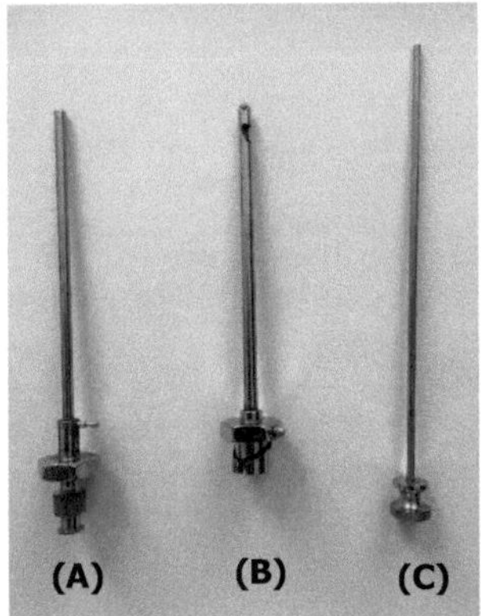

Figure 1: Abrams consisting of three components: A trocar with a lateral opening **(B)** A hollow tube that slides into the trocar **(A)**

A chuck **(C)**

8) Results of pre-therapeutic assessment :

- Liver and kidney function tests, blood count, uricemia

-Ophthalmological examination -HIV serology

9) Treatment regimen :

Treatment regimen: fixed-drug combination (FDC) or dissociated therapy. ADF treatment is when the major anti-tuberculosis drugs are combined in a single capsule **(Table I,II).**

Table I [4]: Antibacterial drugs and their dosages

Drug	Presentation/dosage	Dosage/maximum dose
Rifampicin (R)	300 mg capsule 2% syrup	10mg/kg/d (maximum 600mg/d)
Isoniazid (H)	Tablets (100mg-300mg)	3-5mg/kg/d (maximum 300mg/d)
Pyrazinamide (Z)	Tablets (500mg)	30mg/kg/d (maximum 2000-2500mg/d)
Ethambutol (E)	Tablets (400mg)	20mg/kg/d (maximum 1600-2000mg/d)

Table II [4]: First-line anti-tuberculosis drugs (ADF) and their indications weight-based dosage adults

ADF/Weight	**20-24kg**	**25-29kg**	**30-39kg**	**40-55kg**	**55-70kg**	**>70kg**
HRZE 75mg+150mg+400mg +275mg)	1,5	2	2	3	4	4
HR (75mg+150mg)	1,5	2	2	3	4	4

ADF: fixed drug association

-Treatment duration

- Non-medicinal treatments: pleural puncture, pleural physiotherapy, drainage thoracic

-Therapeutic compliance

Side effects of anti-tuberculosis treatment

10) Evolutionary modalities :

Cure is defined as the absence of any signs clinical and/or laboratory progression.
radiology at the end of anti-tuberculosis treatment [4].

Pleural sequelae are defined by pleural thickening of more than 10mm on the end-of-treatment radiograph on the same side as the initial pleural effusion.

5. Statistical analysis :

For the statistical analysis, data were entered and analyzed using the following software SPSS version 21.

5.1. Descriptive study :

For qualitative variables, simple frequencies and relative frequencies (expressed as percentages) were calculated.

For quantitative variables, averages calculated.

5.2. Analytical study :

Qualitative values were compared using Pearson's chi-square test and Fisher's exact test. A p-value of =<0.05 was chosen as the threshold of significance for our entire statistical study.

6. Bibliographic research :

For the bibliographic search, we used the following keywords: Pleural tuberculosis, epidemiology, treatment, evolution.

The search engines used were : Pubmed - Google scholar - Science direct and Researchgate.

7. Ethical considerations and conflict interest :

Given the retrospective nature of our study, consent was sought. We have no conflicts of interest to declare in this study.

RESULTS

1. General characteristics of the study population

1.1. Frequency :

Fifty cases of pleural TB were recorded during the study period from January 2015 to December 2019, meeting our inclusion and non-inclusion criteria.

Pleural TB accounted for 9.5% of all TB cases reported during the period.

in the CAP BON region **(figure 2)**.

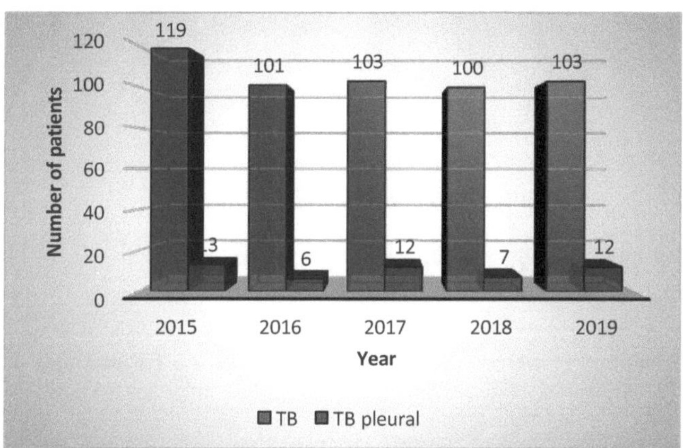

Figure 2: Frequency of pleural tuberculosis in Cap Bon during the period from 2015 to 2019

1.2. Age :

Patient ages ranged from 16 to 89 years, with a mean of 40.4 years, a median of 37 years and a standard deviation of 18.8 years. Over half the patients (62%) were young adults aged between 20 and 50 years **(Figure 3)**.

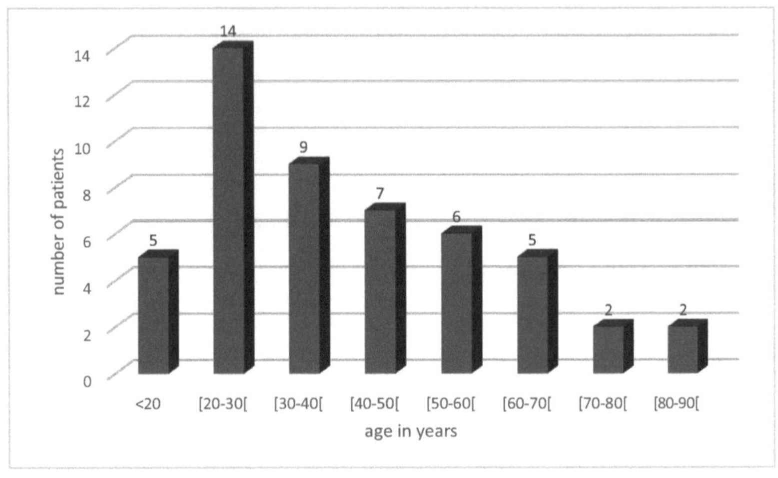

Figure 3: Age of patients

For men, average age 42. For women, it was 36.5.

1.3. Gender :

There were 35 men (70%) and 15 women (30%). The sex ratio was 2.3 **(figure 4)**.

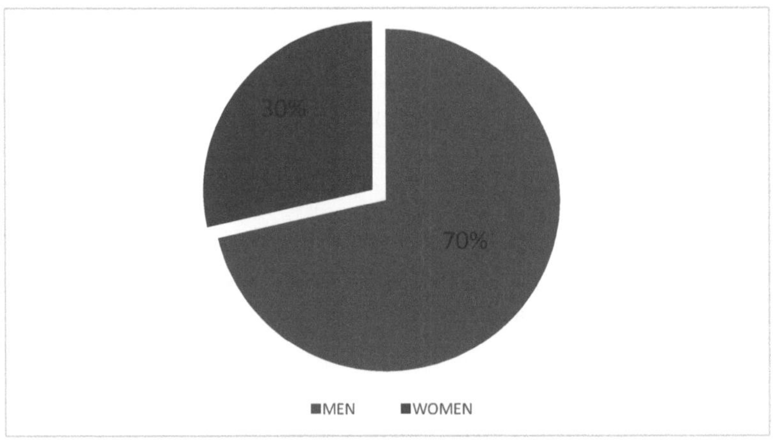

Figure 4: Population distribution by gender

1.4. Geographical origin :

All our patients lived in Tunisia, and came from the CAP BON region, with the Nabeul delegation at the top of the list **(figure 5)**.

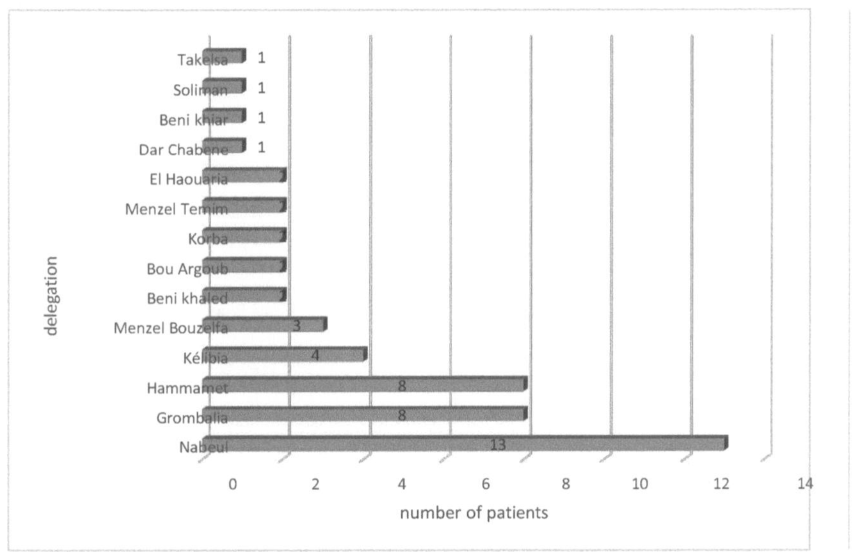

Figure 5: Patient distribution geographic origin

Thirty-eight of our patients (76%) lived in urban areas, and 12 (24%) in rural areas.

1.5. Conditions socio-economic

Occupation was mentioned on the medical records in 44 cases. Twelve patients were unemployed: 6 housewives, 2 retired and 4 unemployed. The majority of the remaining 32 patients were blue-collar workers (50%) (**figure 6**).

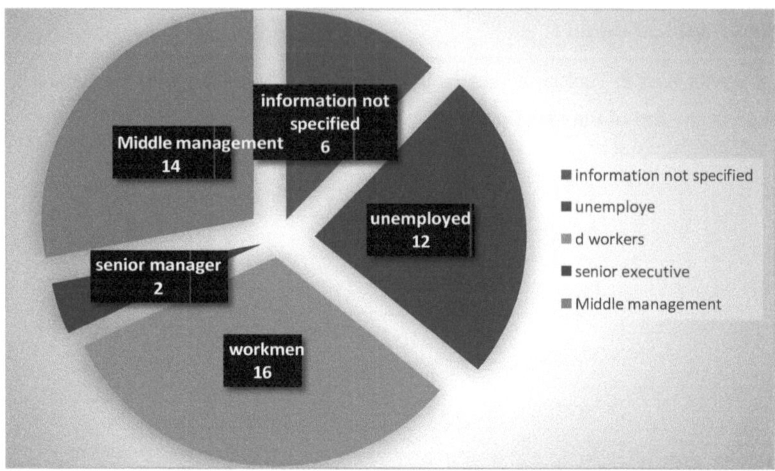

Figure 6: Population distribution by occupation

Educational level was specified in 14 files: 11 patients had a secondary education, 2 had a primary education and only one had acquired a higher education diploma.

An average socio-economic level was noted in 84% of cases (n=44). A good socioeconomic level was noted in 4 cases. Poor socioeconomic status was noted in 2 cases.

Four of our patients had a history of incarceration with a mean age of 35.7 years.

1.6. Pathological history :

1.6.1. Personal history :

Only one patient had a history of pulmonary tuberculosis treated and declared cured in 1980. No cases of resistant tuberculosis were reported.

Tuberculosis infection in the family was found in 8% of cases.

A defect was associated with TB in 11 patients (22%), mainly arterial hypertension (AH) in 7, followed by diabetes in 3 and chronic renal failure in 3, 2 of whom were on hemodialysis. **(figure 7)**.

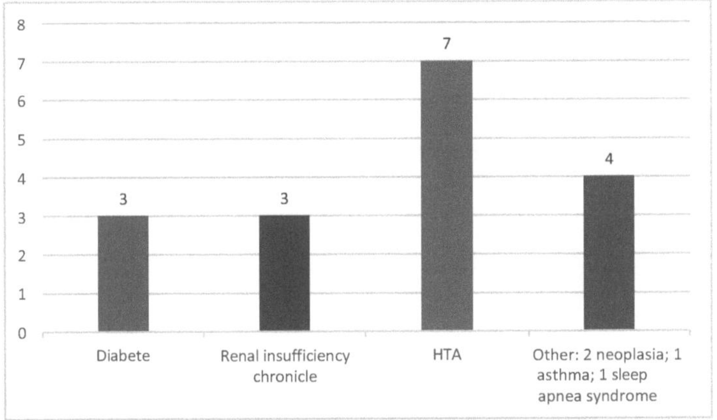

Figure 7: Distribution of patients according to associated defects

Furthermore, none of our patients was on corticosteroid or immunosuppressive therapy.

1.6.2. Family history :

We noted a family history of pulmonary TB in only one case. This involved a first-degree relative who was treated and cured for pulmonary TB.

1.7. BCG vaccination

All patients were vaccinated with BCG

1.8. Habits

1.7.1 Smoking

Twenty-six patients were smokers (52%), with an estimated average consumption of 19 packs a year.

Twenty-one patients were cigarette smokers and 5 were hookah users.

1.7.2 Ethylism and other toxic habits

Eight men were chronic alcohol (16%), and another four
were cannabis smokers, 3 of whom had a history of incarceration.

2. Diagnosis positive

2.1. consultation deadline

The average time onset of clinical signs and consultation was 28 days.
days, with extremes ranging from 4 days to 120 days **(figure 8)**.

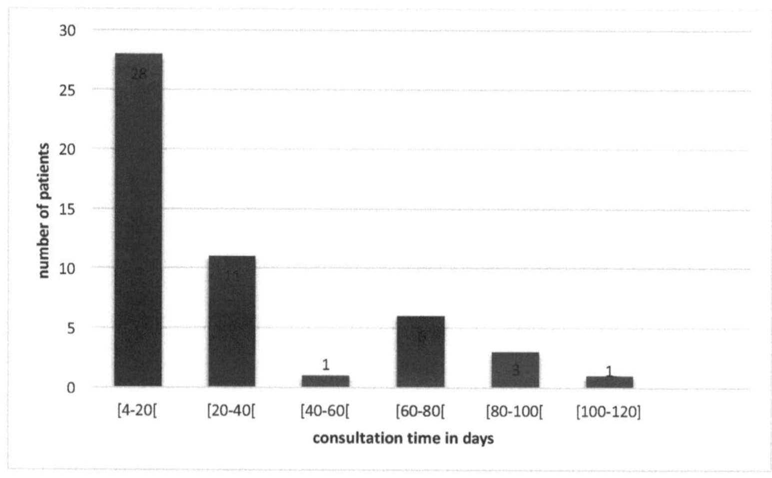

Figure 8: Distribution of patients according to consultation delay

2.2. Clinical signs

2.2.1. Signs respiratory

Respiratory signs were present in all patients. Chest pain was the main symptom reported (80% of cases). This was pleural pain of the side stitch type, aggravated by coughing and changes in position in 9 cases (22%). Cough was reported by 34 patients. Sixteen patients (32%) complained of exertional dyspnea.

2.2.2. Signs

General signs were present in 44 cases (88%), dominated by fever (58% of cases) and night sweats (62% of cases). triad of asthenia, anorexia and weight loss was present in 31 patients (62%) **(Table III)**.

Table III: Population distribution according to clinical signs

Clinical signs	Number of patients	Percentage
Respiratory signs	50	100
Dyspnea	16	32
Cough	34	68
Chest pain	40	80
General signs	44	88
Asthenia-anorexia-weight loss	31	62
Fever	29	58
Sweating	31	62

Examination physical

Fever was present at the time of consultation in 36% of cases (n=18). the majority of cases (92%), a liquid pleural effusion syndrome was noted, with decreased transmission of vocal vibrations on palpation, dullness of the chest on percussion and decreased vesicular murmur on auscultation.

2.3. Biological check-up

CRP elevation above 5 mg/l was noted all cases. Values ranged from 9 to 368 mg/l, with a mean value of 99.5 mg/l.

A predominantly neutrophilic hyperleukocytosis was noted in 7 cases (14%) with a mean value of 14165 elements/mm3, and a microcytic hypochromic anemia in 3 patients (6%).

Lymphopenia was present in 7 patients (14%), with a mean lymphocyte count of 747 cells/mm3. No abnormalities in liver function were noted.

2.4. Check-up radiology

2.4.1. Chest X-ray standard

Chest X-rays revealed a dense, homogeneous pleural opacity that obliterated the costodiaphragmatic angle and extended upwards to form an axillary border line with an upwardly and medially concave boundary in all cases **(figure 9)**.

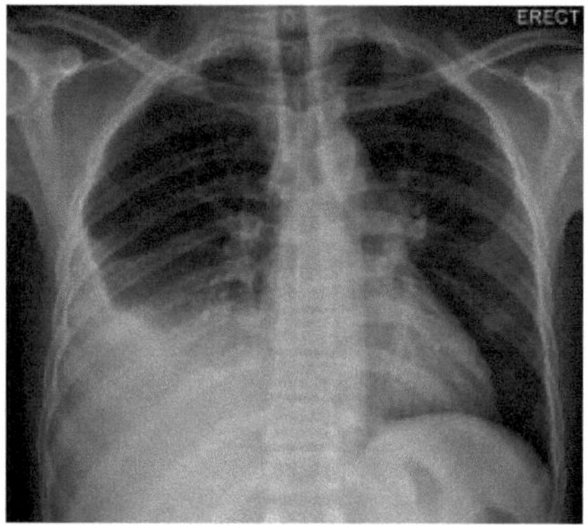

Figure 9: Front chest X-ray showing a dense homogeneous opacity filling the homolateral cul-de-sac and obliterating the diaphragmatic cupola bounded at the top by an italicized S line corresponding to an effusion from the large pleural cavity, probably encysted.

The effusion affected less than one-third of the lung field in 26 patients (52%), and more than one-third in 24 (48%). It was located on the right in 29 patients (58%), on the left in 20 (40%) and bilateral in 1 case. In 5 patients (10%), there were images suggestive of associated progressive pulmonary tuberculosis, in the form of parahilar excavated pulmonary opacities, parenchymal condensations and/or nodular infiltrates predominating at the apices. These images were on the same side as the pleurisy in all cases **(figure 10)**.

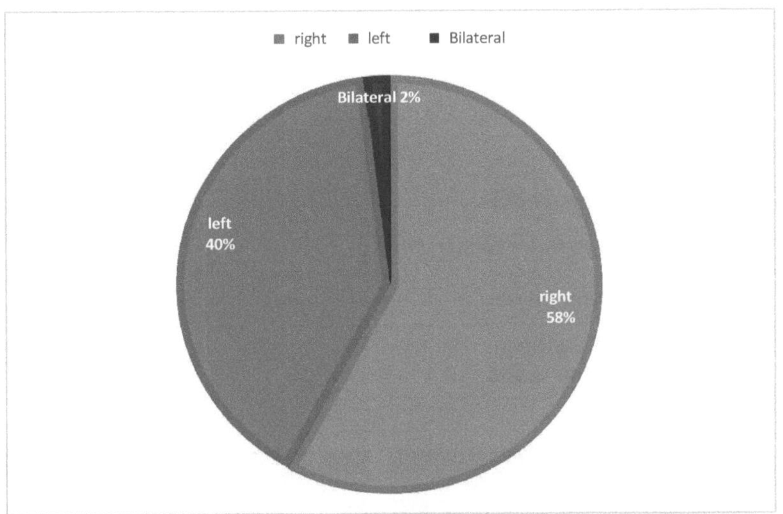

Figure 10: Distribution of patients by location effusion

2.4.2. Ultrasound thoracic

Thoracic ultrasound was performed to guide pleural puncture or biopsy in 42% of cases (n=21). It was indicated after failure of a first exploratory puncture in 9 patients, allowing visualization of partitions in favor encystment, and immediately in the other patients with a small pleural effusion (n=12).

2.4.3. Chest computed tomography (CT)

Chest CT scans were performed in 11 patients (22% of cases). Six patients had had this examination as part of their pre-hospitalization check-up.

Three patients had angio-CT suspected pulmonary embolism during hospitalization, and two patients had chest CT for suspected pleural empyema.

CT signs are summarized in **Table IV** :

Table IV: Chest CT data

	n	Percentage
Free fluid effusion	9	81
Cloisonné effusion	2	18
Mediastinal adenopathy	1	9
Associated pulmonary tuberculosis lesions: subpleural micronodules	1	9
Regular diffuse pleural thickening of the costal	1	9

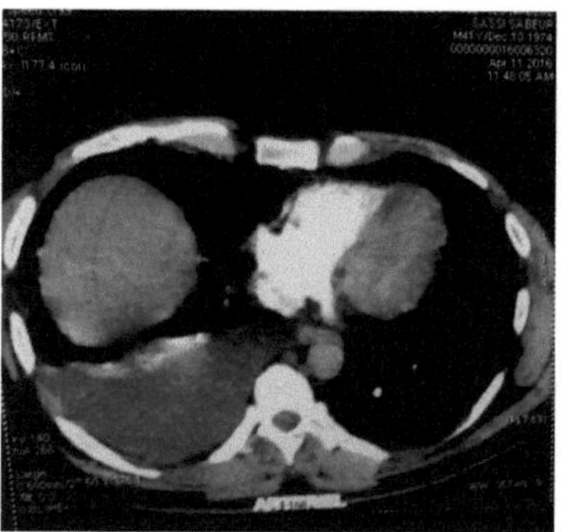

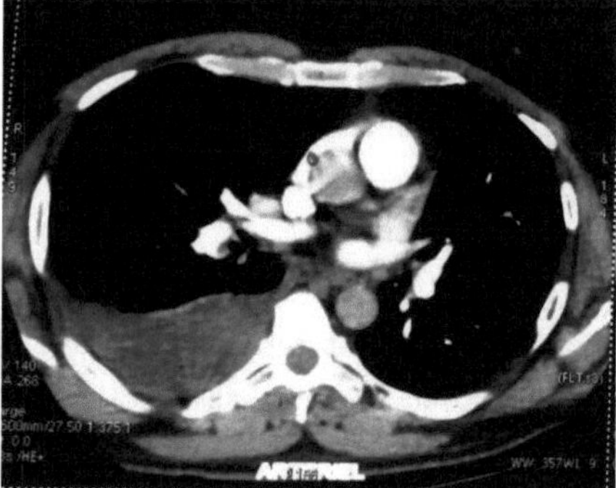

Figure 11: Chest CT scan in axial section and mediastinal window showing a right pleural effusion free of the large cavity.

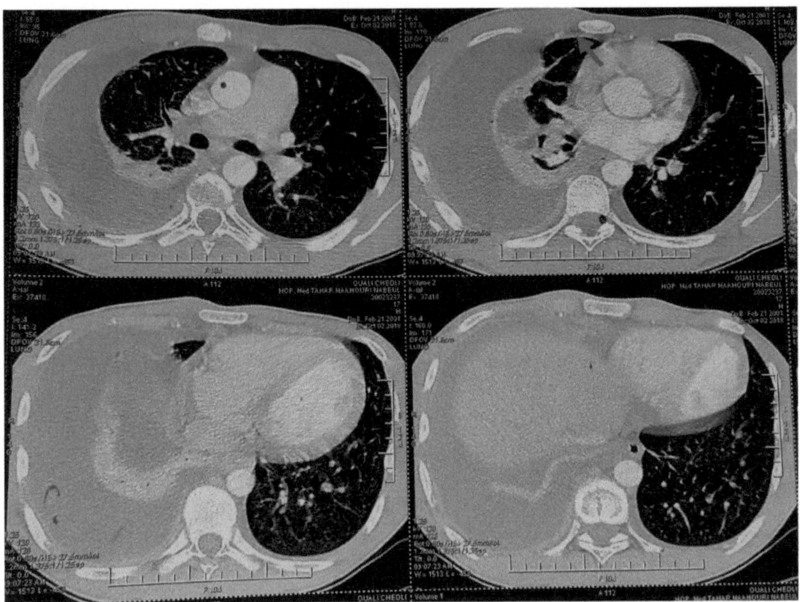

Figure 12: Chest CT scan in axial section and mediastinal window showing a large right pleural effusion associated with regular diffuse right pleural thickening of the costal pleura (red arrow) and non-aerated collapse of the right middle and lower lobes.

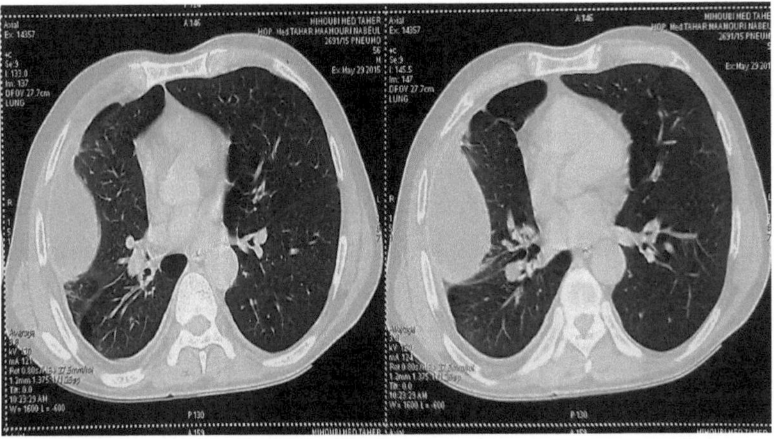

Figure 13: Chest CT scan in axial section and mediastinal window showing an encysted right pleural effusion opposite the middle lobe.

2.5. Intradermal tuberculin reaction

TST was performed in 38 patients (76%). It was positive in 36 patients and negative in 2.

2.6. Confirmatory methods diagnostic

2.6.1. pleural puncture

Pleural puncture was performed in 49 cases. One patient did not have a pleural puncture. pleural nature of his pleurisy.

The appearance of the fluid was citrine yellow in 88% of cases (n=44), cloudy in 4 and hematic in just one.

Pleurisy was exudative in all cases. The mean LP protein level was 53.4 g/l. More than half the patients (64%) had LP protein levels >50g/l.

The mean white blood cell count was 2469 cells/mm3, with lymphocytic predominance in all cases.

Direct examination of pleural puncture fluid for BAARs was positive in one case.

2.6.2. Pleural biopsy (BP)

Blind pleural biopsy with the ABRAMS needle was performed in 47 patients: once in 44 patients, twice in two patients and three times in one patient. The total number of biopsies taken was 51, enabling the diagnosis of pleural TB to be made in 46 cases, giving a cost-effectiveness rate of 90.1%. The average number of biopsy fragments taken was 6.

Complications of blind pleural biopsy were noted in 6 patients: 2 cases of iatrogenic pneumothorax requiring a period of rest and high-concentration mask oxygen therapy at 10-12l/mn, and 4 patients presented with vagal malaise.

Surgical BP per thoracoscopy was performed in 3 patients: immediately in 2 patients with compartmentalized pleurisy and after a single blind non-contributory BP in one patient. The diagnosis was confirmed in all 3 cases.

Anatomopathological study of biopsy fragments revealed a tuberculoid granuloma alone in 24 patients (48%) and associated with caseous necrosis in 25 patients (50%).

2.6.3. Other means of confirmation diagnostic

All patients tested negative for BAARs in sputum, and only one patient tested positive on direct LP examination.

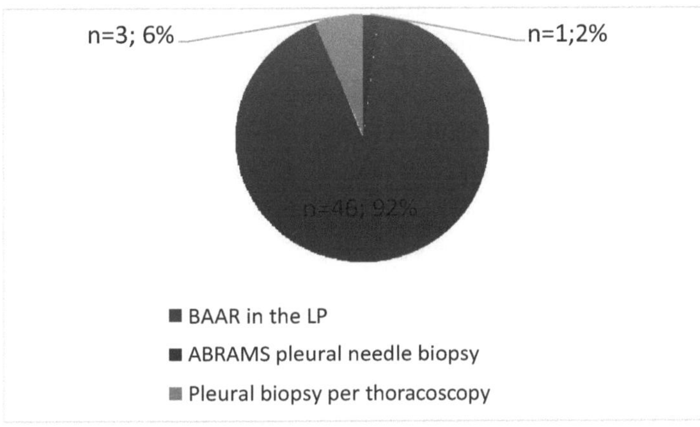

Figure 14: Means of diagnostic confirmation

2.7. Diagnostic delay :

The mean time from onset of symptoms to confirmation of diagnosis was 41.7 days, with extremes ranging from 7 to 127 days. In 13 cases (26%), the delay was more than 60 days.

3. Treatment of tuberculosis pleural

3.1. Treatment

3.1.1. Anti bacillary treatment

3.1.1.1. Pre-treatment assessment

It showed a disturbance of the renal balance in 3 patients known to be carriers. chronic renal failure

A rapid HIV test was performed for all patients with no cases of human immunodeficiency virus co-infection.

An ophthalmological examination was carried out on a single patient as part of the etiological work-up for paroxysmal headaches, and was without anomaly.

3.1.1.2. Initial treatment regimen :

Anti-tuberculosis treatment was carried out in accordance with the recommendations of the national anti-tuberculosis program (PNLT). In the initial phase, a fixed-dose combination of isoniazid, rifampicin, pyrazinamide and ethambutol was prescribed for 46 patients. For the remaining 2 patients, dissociated anti-tuberculosis treatment was indicated due to renal insufficiency (creatinine clearance <25ml/min).

3.1.1.3. Monitoring and compliance

Two of our patients were lost to follow-up: one before the diagnosis was announced and another after initiation of anti-tuberculosis treatment. Another patient was referred back to his home department after diagnostic confirmation. The other patients were reviewed at the consultation: at two weeks after initiation of anti-tuberculosis treatment (47 patients), at 2 months (45 patients, 90%), at 3 months (5 patients, 90%), and at the end of the treatment. patients, 10%), at 4 months (41 patients, 82%), at 5 months (3 patients, 6%) and at 6 months

treatment (47 patients, 94%).

Forty-six patients (92%) showed improvement in general signs after 15 days of treatment. Radiological monitoring was carried out at each consultation for the majority patients. At 2 months after treatment, radiological improvement (reduction in pleural opacity) was achieved in 31 patients (62% of cases), and complete radiological clearance in 9 patients (18% of cases). BAAR testing of control sputum was performed at 2 months after treatment in 4 patients, at 4 months in four patients, at 5 months in two patients and at 6 months in 5 patients. All were negative.

3.1.1.4. Effects

An adverse reaction linked to anti-tuberculosis drugs was found in 7 cases (14%). Two patients presented more than one complication. Two patients presented an allergy to anti-tuberculosis drugs, which was documented by a pharmacovigilance survey.

The average time to onset of side effects was 38.3 days, with extremes ranging from 10 to 70 days **(Table V)**.

Table V: Side effects of anti-tuberculosis drugs

Undesirable effects	n %	Delay in days)	Offending drug	What to do	Therapeutic regimen	Treatment duration
Epigastralgia and/or vomiting	2 4	15	H and R	Symptomatic treatment	2months:HRZE then 4months:H+R	6 months
Arthralgia	1 2	60	Z	Treatment symptomatic	2months:HRZE then 4months:H+R	6 months
Hepatic cytolysis at 10N	2 4	42	H	Discontinuation of anti-tuberculosis treatment until liver function tests normalized, followed by sequential treatment with H with dosage adjustment according to acetylation test, followed by introduction of R		6 months
Isolated pruritus	2 4	60	H	Symptomatic treatment	2months:HRZE then 4months:H+R	6 months
Exanthema maculo- 1 isolated papular	2	70	Z	Arrêt Z and use of 2nd-line antituberculosis drugs: oflocet	2months:HRZE then 4months: R+oflocet	9 months
Maculopapular exanthema with fever	1 2	10	R	Discontinuation of rifampin	3months:H+Z+E then 4months :H+Z	7months

3.1.1.5. Duration of treatment

The duration of treatment was 6 months: 2 months of quadritherapy (Isoniazid, Rifampicin, Pyrazinamide, Ethambutol) followed by 4 months of dual therapy (Isoniazid, Rifampicin) for the majority of patients (44 patients, 88%).

For 3 patients, the therapeutic regimen was extended by 1, 2 and 3 months, for a total treatment duration of 7, 8 and 9 months respectively.

3.2. Non drug treatment

3.2.1. Oxygen therapy

Nine patients (18%) had been placed on oxygen therapy during hospitalization. Oxygen therapy was indicated for large pleural effusions responsible for hypoxemia in 7 patients. Oxygen therapy was weaned after evacuation of the LP.

3.2.2. Physiotherapy pleural

Pleural relaxation physiotherapy was indicated for all patients during hospitalization, and was adhered to by 47 patients (94%).

3.2.3. Evacuation punctures

The LP was evacuated by puncture in 34 patients (68%): The mean number of evacuation punctures was 1 (range 1-3). In only one patient was the LP evacuated by thoracic drainage, due to the compartmentalized nature of the pleurisy.

3.2.4. Pleural decortication surgery

Our patients had no indication for pleural decortication.

3.3. Related measures

3.3.1. Mandatory declaration

All cases of pleural tuberculosis diagnosed in our department were reported.

4. Evolution

Two of our patients were lost to follow-up: one before the diagnosis was announced and another after initiation of anti-tuberculosis treatment. Another patient was referred back to his home department after diagnostic confirmation. For the other patients, cure was declared at the end of anti-tuberculosis treatment in the presence of clinical and radiological improvement.

The average length of follow-up after completion of anti-tuberculosis treatment was 5 months, with extremes ranging from 1 month to 12 months. Four patients were not seen at the consultation after the end of treatment.

Only one patient retained residual basithoracic pain on the side of the pleural effusion. His follow-up chest X-ray was without abnormality. Radiological sequelae were noted by 16 patients (32%) at the end-of-treatment X-ray, with regular pleural thickening in 14 patients and pleural effusion of small volume in 2 patients.

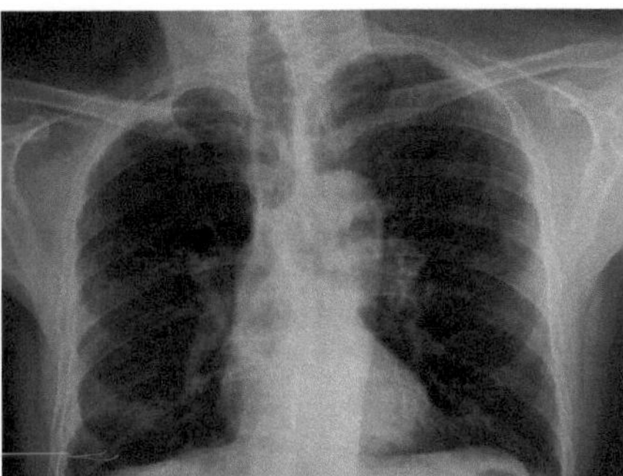

Figure 15: Frontal chest X-ray at the end of anti-tuberculosis treatment showing sequelae of apical pleural thickening.

No statistically significant association between the appearance of pleural sequelae and the following parameters: active smoking, presence of parenchymal lesions on the initial radiograph, sex, age, time to consultation with respective p values of 0.6; 0.2; 0.9; 0.4; 0.7 and 0.8.

DISCUSSION

TB remains a major cause of morbidity and mortality worldwide, particularly in developing countries. Tunisia is a country with intermediate TB endemicity. Extra-pulmonary involvement accounted for 62% of all TB cases in 2017, with a steady increase in its frequency in recent years, particularly with regard to lymph node and pleural TB [4]. The latter form is poorly described in the literature, and its diagnosis is often difficult due to the paucibacillary nature of bacteriological specimens. In this context, we carried out a retrospective descriptive study of

50 records of pleural TB patients managed in the Pneumology Department Mohamed Taher Maamouri Hospital over a 4-year period (January 2015 - December 2019).

The objectives of our work were to :

-describe the epidemiological profile of pleural TB in Cap Bon

-identify its clinical features

-specify its therapeutic and evolutionary modalities

Our population comprised 35 men (70%) and 15 women (30%). The mean age was 40.4 years. No patient was HIV-positive, 7 patients were hypertensive, 3 patients were diabetic and 3 others had chronic renal failure, 2 of whom were hemodialysis. The average consultation time was 28 days.

Respiratory symptoms were reported by all patients, dominated by chest pain (80% of cases) and dyspnoea (32% of cases). General signs were present in 88% of cases. Pleurisy was right-sided in 58% of cases, and parenchymal involvement was associated with 5 patients.

ABRAMS pleural needle biopsy confirmed the diagnosis of pleural TB in 46 cases. Direct examination of the LP for BAARs was positive in one patient. Thoracoscopic pleural biopsy confirmed the diagnosis of pleural TB in 3 patients.

The evolution of pleural tuberculosis under well-administered anti-tuberculosis treatment was favorable, with a cure rate of 94%. Sixteen patients had radiological sequelae of pleural thickening or residual pleural effusion.

Like all scientific work, ours has a number of strengths and weaknesses. It's true that pleural TB is a topical issue, and its incidence is increasing in our country, but few Tunisian studies have focused on the subject. Knowledge of its various radio-clinical presentations, as well as its different diagnostic and therapeutic modalities, therefore seems essential.

Another strong point worth noting is that the study period enabled us to look back 4 years and therefore evaluate the follow-up of our patients.

What's more, in our current practice, a consultation every Friday is dedicated to tuberculosis patients, ensuring better organization of patient follow-up. During this consultation, patients receive a clinical evaluation and, in some cases, a biological or radiological work-up.

The main limitation of our study is its retrospective nature, with some clinical and paraclinical data lost or missing.

The frequency of pleural TB varies from study to study and from country to country. It is the second most common form of extra-pulmonary tuberculosis, after lymph node involvement [4, 9, 10]. It accounts for less than 1% of all exudative effusions in Western countries, occurring in only 3 to 5% of TB patients (5.9% in New Zealand; 5.6% in the) [11], it is responsible for

30 to 80% of all pleural effusions encountered in developing countries such as India, and can complicate tuberculosis in 31% of cases [12]. It is the leading cause of clear-fluid pleurisy in Madagascar (70.28%) [13], Burkina-Faso (63.15%) [14] and Côte d'Ivoire (66%) [15]. In these countries with a high prevalence of tuberculosis, this diagnosis should be considered in all patients presenting with pleurisy of undetermined etiology [6].

Its frequency is higher in African countries where HIV prevalence is high (>20% of all forms of tuberculosis) [16] while in the the figure is 5% [10].

In our country, pleural localization is one of the most frequent sites of TBEP. It ranked first in the series by Zorai [5] and Ben Ghars [17], accounting for 52% and 40% of TBEP respectively. In a study carried out in the Sousse region, pleural localization ranked second after lymph node localization, accounting for 17.6% of TBEP [18].

Pleural TB can affect all age groups, but adults are most at risk, especially during the productive years of their lives. In fact, this age group is often socially active, frequenting a greater or lesser number of people at work or play, thus increasing the likelihood of contagion [1].

Similarly, in our study, the average age of our population 40.4 +/- 18.8 years, and over half of our patients (62%) were young adults aged between 20 and 50 years. These results are similar to those found in the literature. Thus, in Bemba's series [10] and Ouardi's series

[19], patients had an average age of 39 and 44 respectively. Similarly, Ajmi [18] revealed in his work that pleural tuberculosis mainly affects (70% of cases) young adults aged between 15 and 44. Table VII summarizes the average age of pleural TB patients in different countries **(Table VI)**.

Table VI: Average age of pleural TB patients in different countries

Series	Country/City	Year	Average age (years)
Bemba [10]	Congo/Brazzaville	2017	39
Ouardi [19]	Morocco/Marrakech	2016	44
Perfura Yone [20]	Cameroon/Yaoundé	2011	36,7
Aazri [21]	Morocco/Marrakech	2018	36
Ben Ghars [17]	Tunisia	2007	33
Our series	Tunisia/Cape Bon	2019	40,42

To a lesser extent, tuberculosis can affect the elderly population, particularly in countries with a low prevalence of TB disease. In this context, it is sometimes due to the evolution of a recent infection, but above all to the reactivation of a latent infection favoured by the ageing of the immune system and also by comorbidities, notably diabetes and renal failure, which are frequently associated in this age group [9, 22, 23].

Poor socio-economic conditions are recognized as a factor in the spread of transmissible infectious diseases in general, and tuberculosis in particular, especially in its extra-pulmonary form. , the insalubrious living conditions, malnutrition and promiscuity can only facilitate the spread this contagious disease. On the other hand, the difficulty of access to medical care due to poverty and the frequent absence of social security coverage is often the cause of delays in consultation and diagnosis [24, 25]. This was clearly demonstrated in our study, where half the patients were blue-collar workers, an often impoverished social category.

Moreover, a higher prevalence of TBEP has been observed in unemployed patients [26]. This was also the case in our population: 25% of patients (12 patients) were unemployed.

Extra-pulmonary tuberculosis, in this case pleural tuberculosis, is more likely affect subjects with weak immune defenses. HIV co-infection is a factor of immunodepression, well studied in the literature, favoring the extra-pulmonary spread of this infection. Thus, since the emergence of HIV infection in the 1980s, the proportion of TBEP cases relative to the number of tuberculosis cases in general has increased. In the United States, for example, this proportion has risen from 15% in 1978 to 60% in people living with HIV, of whom 30% have only extra-pulmonary TB and 30% have PPT associated with pulmonary TB [27]. In sub-Saharan Africa, the region of the world most affected by HIV, this proportion is also high, reaching 50% of cases according to a study carried out in TOGO in 2017 [28].

In Tunisia, prevalence of HIV infection is low, around 0.016% in 2018.
[29] and its impact on tuberculosis is minor [4]. Nevertheless, the Tunisian national tuberculosis control program recommends systematic screening for HIV co-infection in all tuberculosis patients, in order to be able to make the right decision in terms of treatment and monitoring of this disease [4]. In our study, no patient was HIV-positive.

In patients with chronic renal failure undergoing hemodialysis, tuberculosis is frequently extra-pulmonary, accounting for up to 71% of cases. , immunosuppression caused by chronic uraemia favours extra-pulmonary dissemination of tuberculosis infection [30].

The consultation delay is the time between the onset of clinical signs and the date of the first medical consultation. In our study, this delay was 28 days. This result is comparable to another Tunisian study carried out in La Marsa (27.8 days).
[17] and shorter than that reported in Cherif's series (43.6 days) [31].

Several parameters determine the delay in consultation. On the one hand, there are the characteristics of the disease itself; indeed, an insidious onset of symptoms, as is frequently the case with pleural TB, is often responsible for delayed consultation. On the other hand, the characteristics of the healthcare system, notably ease of access to medical care, have a strong influence on this delay. In developing countries, such as Nigeria (12.3 weeks on average) and South Africa (10 weeks) [32, 33], consultation times are longer, whereas they are shorter in developed countries such as Hong Kong (20 days) [34].

Pleural TB may be completely asymptomatic and be discovered by chance on a chest X-ray taken an employment or premarital check-up, but in the majority of cases it is suspected by the association of general signs and respiratory signs of dyspnea and pleural pain of insidious evolution [12].

All our patients had respiratory symptoms at the time of diagnosis, dominated by chest pain in 80% of , followed by cough in 68% and exertional dyspnoea in 32%. General signs were present in most of our patients (88%), with fever in 58% of cases and night sweats in 62%.

In a retrospective study of 228 patients in Morocco, Ouardi found that the most frequent symptoms were chest pain, dyspnoea and cough, observed in 88.3, 77.3 and 82.2% of cases respectively [17].

According to a literature review published in 2018, the most common symptoms were fever (in 75% of cases)pleural-type chest pain (50-75% of cases) and a non-productive cough in 70-75% of cases. Other symptoms described were exertional dyspnea in 50% of cases, and general signs such as night sweats and weight loss (respectively 50% and 25-85% of cases). [22] **(Table VII)**.

Table VII: Prevalence of each clinical sign in different series

Reference	Chest pain (%)	Cough (%)	Dyspnea (%)	Fever (%)	AEG (%)	Night sweats (%)
Perfura Yone **(Cameroon 2011) [20]**	88,6	78,9	71,9	74,6	84,2	43,9
Ouardi (Morocco 2016) [19]	88,3	82,2	77,3	-	-	-
Ketata (Tunisia) 2014) [2]	77,5	94	-	86	-	-
Aazri (Morocco 2018) [21]	78,7	85	73,7	61,2	75	55
Our series	80	68	32	58	62	62

Radiologically, tuberculous pleural effusion is most often unilateral and variable in size, affecting more than two-thirds of a hemithorax in 18.5% of cases, between one-third and two-thirds of the lung field in almost half of cases, and less than one-third of a hemithorax in 34% of cases [12, 22].

In our seriespleural effusion was unilateral in 98% of cases, of low to moderate abundance in half the cases, affecting less than a third of the lung field, and in other half of great abundance, affecting more a third of the hemithorax.

No radiological sign is specific for pleural tuberculosis, but certain lesions may point to associated pulmonary involvement and suggest the tuberculous origin of the effusion. These include excavated lesions or nodular or micronodular infiltrates predominating in the upper lobes [35]. In our study, 10% of patients had radiological lesions suggestive of associated pulmonary tuberculosis: these excavated pulmonary opacities para hilar, de condensations parenchymatous et d'infiltrats nodulaires predominant at the summits.

On thoracic ultrasonography, tuberculous pleurisy often presents free anechogenic fluid within the pleural cavity. However, encysted and/or compartmentalized pleurisy or echogenic fluid suggestive of empyema are also possible [7, 22, 36].

Thoracic ultrasound is also useful for guiding diagnostic pleural sampling. It is recommended by the British Thoracic Society (BTS) to guide pleural puncture in cases of small effusion or after failure of a first blind pleural puncture. However, given its safety and the ease with which it can be performed at the patient's bedside, pleural puncture should be performed systematically prior to any pleural sampling. This reduces the risk of complications and increases the cost-effectiveness of the procedure, particularly blind BP, by localized pleural thickening or pleural nodules [7, 37]. Young respirologists in training should therefore be encouraged learn this technique.

In our study, it was indicated in 21 patients. In 9 cases, it was requested after failure of a first blind exploratory puncture. For these patients, it revealed intra-pleural septations. In the other patients, it was performed to guide puncture in the presence of a small pleural effusion.

Thoracic CT is currently considered the best imaging modality for visualizing the pleura and lung parenchyma in pleural tuberculosis, but is not routinely performed. It is indicated in cases of diagnostic doubt or suspicion of complications such as pleural empyema. This is suggested on imaging by the presence of a sub pleural abscess or broncho pleural fistula [7, 36].

Computed tomography is superior to standard chest radiography in detecting associated parenchymal lesions. According to a recent review of the literature, the frequency of such lesions can be as high as 80% of cases, compared with 20-50% on standard chest radiography. The most frequent parenchymal abnormalities subpleural and peribronchovascular micronodules, pleural thickening and parenchymal condensations [22, 38].

In a study by Kim et al including 106 patients with pleural TB, associated parenchymal lesions were visualized in 91 of the patients (86% of cases) on chest CT [38].

In our study, 11 patients underwent thoracic CT, 5 of them during hospitalization: three for suspected pulmonary embolism and two for suspected pleural empyema. Chest CT revealed parenchymal abnormalities such as subpleural micronodules and pleural thickening, undetected on chest X-ray in 2 patients.

In recent years, a number of biomarkers have been developed to help diagnose pleural TB, particularly in difficult cases where conventional bacteriological and/or histological investigations have proved inconclusive. These include immunobiochemical markers such as interferon-gamma (IFN), adenosine deaminase 2 (ADA2) isoenzyme and total adenosine deaminase (ADA), and molecular biological markers such as the Xpert MTB/RIF polymerase chain reaction (PCR) and the interferon-gamma release assay (IGRA) [7, 40].

In the absence of associated parenchymal lesions suggestive of TB, BAAR testing spontaneous sputum is not very cost-effective for the diagnosis of pleural TB, with a sensitivity of around 4-7% [41]. It is, however, more useful in patients suffering from immunosuppression secondary to HIV co-infection [40, 42].

Some studies have looked at the contribution of induced sputum to the diagnosis of pleural TB in the absence of associated radiological lung lesions. This is sputum obtained after nebulization with 5% hypertonic salfor 10 to 20 minutes using an ultrasonic nebulizer [43]. Conde et al, in their prospective study of 113 patients, found a 55% yield from the culture of these induced sputum [44]. However, this technique is likely to increase the risk of contamination of nursing staff [45].

All our patients were tested for BAARs in spontaneous sputum, and all came back negative.

Pleural puncture is an easy, routine procedure in pneumology. It enables the macroscopic and microscopic characteristics of the effusion be determined, and sometimes confirms the diagnosis of pleural TB by demonstrating BAARs on direct examination and/or Mycobacterium tuberculosis on LP culture [42].

According to a review of the literature published in 2015, pale yellow coloration of the LP is the most frequent, found in 80% of cases [7]. This agrees with the data from our study, and a citrine yellow appearance of the LP was found in 88% of cases.

The effusion in tuberculous pleurisy is exudative, with a pleural protide level in the LP> 35gr/l and a pleural protide/blood protide ratio> 0.5 [45]. In the case of pleural protide levels between 25 and 35 gr/l, light criteria can be used to correct the diagnosis of exudate [7]. In 50% of cases, LP protide levels may exceed 50 g/l [7, 35, 46].

Glycopleuria is usually low, between 3.3 and 5.6 mmol/L. Glycopleuria of less than 3.3 mmol/L (0.6 gr/L) should raise concern about associated empyema [10, 39].

The level of lactate dehydrogenase (LDH) in the LP is generally higher than its blood level, often exceeding 500 IU/l. In a series of 77 patients with pleural TB, Groote-Bidlingmaier et al found a mean intrapleural LDH level of 947±1425 IU/l [50]. The PH is often lower than 7.4, of the order of 7.30 [35, 40].

In our study, all patients had an exudative LP with a mean protide level of 53.4 g/l. More than half the patients (64%) (n=32) had protidopleuria >50g/l. LDH measurement in LP and glycopleuria measurement were not performed in our study.

In our current practice, pleural LDH is not routinely measured. It is reserved for cases of diagnostic doubt as to whether pleurisy is transudative or exudative, with a pleural protein level of between 25 and 35 gr/l. In this case, a pleural LDH/blood LDH ratio> of 0.6 confirms the exudative nature of the effusion, with reference to Light's criteria [48].

In the case of pleural TB, the LP cell count is hypercellular, with nucleated elements ranging from 1000 to 6000 cells/ml. Lymphocyte predominance is often found. This is defined by a pleural lymphocyte count of over 50% of all nucleated elements, which may exceed 90%, or by a lymphocyte/neutrophil (PNN) ratio in the LP >0.5. A predominance of neutrophils can, however, be observed in the first two weeks of the infectious process [35, 48, 49].

In our study, lymphocyte predominance LP was found in all cases, with a mean lymphocyte count of 83.5%.

Pleural TB is often paucibacillary, and direct examination of the LP after Ziel-Nielsen staining detects BAARs in only 10% of cases. In patients living HIV, this percentage is higher, to 20% of cases [42, 50]. Culture is more sensitive, being positive in 12 to 70% of cases [51].

The use of liquid media and automated reading systems such as the Bactec system improves culture sensitivity and shortens Mycobacterium tuberculosis detection times (between 7 and 12 days) [52].

Pleural biopsy helps establish the diagnosis of tuberculosis pleurisy by demonstrating, anatomopathological examination of biopsy fragments, an epithelioid and giganto-cellular granuloma associated or not with caseous necrosis, which is found in 50 to 97% of cases, or on microbiological examination of these fragments after culture on Lowenstein Jensen medium of Mycobacterium tuberculosis. Combining histological and bacteriological examination of pleural biopsies, the diagnostic yield can reach 60-95% [40].

Castelman or Abrams needle pleural biopsy has been the most widely used technique over the last 5 decades. Initially described by De Francis in 1955, the biopsy needle was improved in 1958 by Abrams, Cope and Castellin in 1964, and in 1998 by Christian Boutin (1933-2015). The trocar is inserted through the skin into the pleura. A small fragment

pleura is inserted through the side window of the trocar, and the tube sliding into the trocar guillotines the pleura fragment. The internal mandrel seals the system [8].
While this technique is increasingly being abandoned in wealthy countries in favour of surgical techniques, it is still widely used in developing countries.

This is because of the many advantages it offers, notably its low cost and accessibility, making it possible to avoid having to resort to surgery which is sometimes unavailable in certain hospitals. In addition, the technique is simple to perform and easy for young pulmonologists in training to learn. Its cost-effectiveness depends not only on the operator's experience, but also on the thickness of the pleura, the abundance of effusion, the number of fragments removed and the extent of the lesions. It was around 65% in the series by Toloba et al [53]. The use ultrasound or thoracic CT to detect localized pleural thickening improves sensitivity, reaching 90%. There are no data in the literature on the optimal number of biopsy fragments to be taken, but according to Kirsch et al, the diagnostic sensitivity of BP is best when at least 6 fragments are taken [54]. Its main limitation is the blind nature of the biopsy samples and narrowness of the fragments, which are no more than a few millimetres in size. However, a thoracic ultrasound scan to detect localized pleural thickening or pleural nodules can easily overcome this drawback [7, 37]. Complications are rare and mild, with iatrogenic pneumothorax being the most common, rarely requiring pleural evacuation, and usually resolving within a few days with conservative measures combining bed rest and high-concentration mask oxygen therapy (10-12 l/min), as in the case of our two patients [53]. One problem that be raised is the current unavailability of biopsy forceps, which are being manufactured less and less. Local production of this needle should be considered by the health authorities, particularly as it a simple device to manufacture.

Thoracoscopic pleural biopsy is the technique of first resort for the diagnosis of lymphocytic pleurisy of undetermined etiology in developed countries, whereas its use is not first-line in developing countries due to its high cost.

In our context, it is indicated if bacteriological samples are negative, and if blind BP is non-contributory, or if it is not feasible due to a contraindication linked to the patient's condition (haemostasis disorder, poor cooperation), or due to the compartmentalized nature of the effusion preventing blind biopsies. Classically, two BPs are often recommended indicating surgical thoracoscopy [55]. The sensitivity of surgical pleural biopsy is of the order of 100%, but it is associated with more complications and longer hospital stays than blind BP [7, 16,

22, 34, 56, 57].

In our study, needle BP was carried out 51 times, and was used establish the diagnosis of pleural TB in 46 cases, giving a cost-effectiveness rate of 90.1%.

The Mycobacterium tuberculosis polymerase chain reaction is a molecular biology technique based on the amplification of a specific mycobacterial DNA sequence in sufficient numbers to be detectable.

The best-studied genes are IS6110, GCRS, MPB-64, devR CD192, with variable sensitivity and specificity [58]. This is a rapid technique, enabling a response to be obtained within a few hours. A meta-analysis including 14 studies, carried out in countries with a low prevalence of TB, found a sensitivity of 62% and a specificity of 98% for PCR in LP for the diagnosis of tuberculous pleurisy [59].

The GeneXpert system is a fully automated real-time PCR system that does not require a molecular biology laboratory. The Xpert MTB/RIF test has been recommended by the WHO since 2010. It can be used to screen for both tuberculosis and resistance to rifampin and isoniazid. It is a rapid test (results obtained in two hours) that is more sensitive than microscopy (sensitivity over 95% when direct examination of respiratory samples is positive, and around 65 and 77% when this examination is negative). Specificity is high, ranging from 97% to 100%.

The Xpert MTB/RIF Ultra test is even more sensitive than the Xpert MTB/RIF test. It is able to detect very low concentrations of mycobacteria, making it more suitable for use in children and people living with HIV, who often have pauci bacillary forms of tuberculosis. In 2020, the WHO is recommending the use of rapid molecular tests as a universal test to replace microscopic examination of smears [60]. However, these tests remain costly, which limits their use, particularly in low-income countries such ours [40].

Interferon gamma release assays (IGRA) are performed in vitro on a blood sample or on the LP. They measure the release of interferon gamma by T lymphocytes after stimulation with Mycobacterium Tuberculosis antigens [61]. Two tests are marketed: Quantiferon-TB Gold in tube, Quantiferon-TB Gold Plus by ELISA and T-SPOT TB. These tests are more specific than tuberculin skin tests due to the absence of cross-reactivity with BCG and many non-tuberculous mycobacteria. They identify patients infected with Mycobacterium Tuberculosis, but cannot differentiate between latent and diseased tuberculosis, or between old and new tuberculosis infections [4]. They are therefore of little use in diagnosing tuberculous pleurisy [40].

Adenosine deaminase is ubiquitous enzyme involved in the metabolism of purine bases, widely found in T lymphocytes. Several studies have confirmed the value of the ADA assay in LP as a simple, inexpensive means of diagnosing tuberculous pleurisy, with a sensitivity of around 92%, a specificity of and a cut-off value of 44 IU/L. False positives include HIV co-infection and purulent or para-pneumonic pleurisy. In the latter two cases, the lymphocyte formula of the LP can be used to correct the diagnosis of pleural tuberculosis. The main limitation of this biochemical marker is the absence of microbiological documentation, preventing the detection any resistance to anti-tuberculosis drugs in the event of treatment failure [40, 62]. Determination of this enzyme is not available in Tunisia.

adenosine deaminase 2 isoenzyme accounts for 88% of total ADA observed in pleural tuberculosis. Its determination would therefore be more cost-effective than total ADA for the diagnosis of tuberculous pleurisy. However, few studies have evaluated the value of this marker, and its determination is not standard practice [63].

Interferon gamma is a cytokine produced by CD4 T lymphocytes. It increases the bactericidal activity of macrophages against Mycobacterium tuberculosis and is involved in granuloma formation. Several studies have demonstrated the increase in intra-pleural INF gamma levels during tuberculous pleurisy. The sensitivity of this assay has been estimated at 78% to 100%, and its specificity at 95% to . However, the high cost of this assay limits its use in routine practice [64].

Other biomarkers are of interest in the diagnosis of pleural TB, such as C-reactive protein, whose level above 50 mg/l in LP would be in favor of the tuberculous origin of lymphocytic pleurisy with a specificity of 95%, whereas a level <30 mg/l has a specificity of 95% to exclude the diagnosis [65]. A few studies have demonstrated elevated levels of interleukin 6 (IL-6), interleukin 1 alpha (IL-1α) and tumor necrosis factor alpha (TNF-α) in LP during tuberculous pleurisy. These markers are little studied and their place in the diagnosis of tuberculous pleurisy remains to be established [66].

The natural course of pleural TB may be towards spontaneous resolution after 4 to 16 weeks, but with a risk of development of pulmonary or extra-pulmonary tuberculosis in 43-65% of cases [18, 67]. Treatment is aimed at preventing further development of active tuberculosis, relieving symptoms and avoiding pleural sequelae [12]. The regimen of antituberculosis chemotherapy for pleural tuberculosis is the same as for pulmonary tuberculosis. In Tunisia, the protocol adopted is that recommended by the PNLT, whose principles are taken from WHO guidelines updated in 2017 [4, 68].

The recommended treatment regimen for a new case of pleural TB, in the absence of any documented bacterial resistance, consists of a combination of four essential first-line anti-tuberculosis drugs: Isoniazid, Rifampicin, Pyrazinamide and Ethambutol. It comprises two successive phases:

- An initial or intensive phase lasting two months, during which the patient receives the four first-line HRZE anti-tuberculosis drugs on a daily basis. This phase serves to rapidly destroy tubercle bacilli, prevent the emergence of resistance and limit contagiousness.

- A maintenance phase lasting 4 months, during which the patient receives two drugs (HR combination) every day. This phase serves to eliminate the remaining Mycobacterium Tuberculosis bacilli and sterilize the lesions.

Medication must be taken in the morning on an empty stomach at least 30 minutes before any food intake, and under the direct supervision of a health-care staff member or family member: this is the TOD (treatment under direct supervision) strategy. This strategy is recommended by the PNLT to ensure good therapeutic adherence, thus reducing the risk of acquired drug resistance, therapeutic failure, relapse or poor results.

The WHO recommends the use of fixed-dose combinations of anti-tuberculosis drugs. This limits prescription errors and ensures better compliance by reducing the number of tablets to be ingested by the patient.

In the event of documented resistance to first-line anti-tuberculosis drugs, it is recommended that the patient be referred to a center specializing in the treatment of multidrug-resistant tuberculosis (MDR-TB), in order to prescribe second-line anti-tuberculosis drugs [4].

Given the pauci bacillary nature of pleural TB, some teams have proposed simpler treatment regimens. Canete et al. adopted a therapeutic protocol based on Isoniazid and Rifampicin for 6 months, which enabled them to achieve cure without recurrence after three years of follow-up in a series of 130 patients [69]. For the team of Dutt et al, only one therapeutic failure was observed with this same protocol, while cure was obtained for 161 patients without recurrence up to 133 months of follow-up [70]. Other teams have proposed a 9-month treatment with Iisoniazide and rifampicin if the organisms are fully sensitive to the drug [16].

However, these treatment regimens can only be applied in regions with low levels of bacterial resistance [67].

In our series, the proposed treatment followed the recommendations of the NTP. cases of MDR-TB were documented. A second-line anti-tuberculosis drug was used in only one case, due to an allergy to Isoniazid and Pyrazinamide. In this case, the duration of treatment was extended to 9 months. For another patient, the duration of treatment was extended to 7 months due to intolerance to Rifampicin. This patient received 3 months Isoniazid, Pyrazinamide, Ethambutol and 4 months Isoniazid with Pyrazinamide.

Isolation is indicated only for bacilliferous patients [22].

Corticosteroid therapy is not proposed by the NTP for the treatment of pleural TB. Some authors have associated it with the initial phase of anti-tuberculosis treatment, to its anti-inflammatory effect, at a dose of 0.75 to 1 mg/kg/day of prednisone equivalent for a duration of 4 to 12 weeks. They observed a rapid resolution of general signs, however, there was no statically significant difference regarding the development of pleural sequelae [70-72].

A Cochrane review published in 2007 does not support the use of systemic corticosteroids for the treatment of pleural tuberculosis [74]. However, in certain patients suffering from intense general signs (fever, pleural pain, altered general condition), the administration of a short course of corticosteroids at dose of 80 mg/day until the initial clinical signs have disappeared prove useful [16, 67].

Evacuation of pleural effusion should be considered in cases of poor clinical tolerance. It is usually performed by evacuation puncture. It provides rapid relief of dyspnea, improves ventilatory mechanics and prevents sequelae of pleural thickening [22, 67]. Bhuniya et al compared the evolution of pleural TB at six months between a first group receiving anti-tuberculosis treatment combined with pleural evacuation and a second receiving anti-tuberculosis treatment alone. They observed a better gain in forced vital capacity and forced expiratory volume in the first group and less sequellar pleural thickening [75]. However, the long-term consequences of complete pleural evacuation remain unknown.

[22, 67].

Some authors have studied the benefits of thoracic drainage with intrapleural instillation of a fibrolysing agent in cases of compartmentalized tuberculous pleurisy. They have observed an acceleration in the time to resorption of pleural effusion and a reduction in the risk of sequelae of pleural thickening [76, 77].

Thoracic drainage is necessary in cases of tuberculous poypneumothorax, enabling closure of the bronchopleural fistula [78].

In our studypleural evacuation was carried out by evacuation puncture in 68% of cases (n= 34), and by drainage in a single patient with pleurisy of great abundance after failure of pleural puncture attempts. In the Tunisian series by Kmis, 15 patients (33%) required repeated pleural punctures [5]. In the series by Horo et al, pleural drainage was indicated for hydropneumothorax and pneumothorax in 15.2% of cases [79].

Any pleural effusion should be treated systematically with respiratory rehabilitation. It helps limit functional sequelae by improving bronchial drainage and maintaining pulmonary expansion. It also prevents the formation thick, rigid adhesions by promoting LP resorption [80].

In patients treated for pleural TB, the frequency of residual pleural opacity≥ 10 mm at the end of anti-tuberculosis treatment was 22% in the series by Balkissou et al. In this series, 74% of patients had received respiratory physiotherapy during the intensive phase of treatment. This percentage was higher in the study by Han et al (50.6%), in which patients received anti-tuberculosis treatment alone [81,82].

Physiotherapy was indicated during hospitalization for all our patients, and was adhered to by 47 patients.

Since the advent of anti-tuberculosis drugs, the role of surgery in the treatment of thoracic tuberculosis in general, and pleural TB in particular, has become increasingly limited, and is currently confined to the treatment of sequelae [83].

Pleural decortication can be proposed for infected pleural pockets that have been chronic for more than three months, or that are extensive (occupying more than 25% of the pleural cavity) and associated with functional impairment. This technique is used to eliminate these pockets, thereby freeing the lung improving its ventilatory mechanics. Thoracotomy remains the standard technique for decortication, although video-thoracoscopy is becoming increasingly important, offering the advantage of shorter hospital stays and a lower complication rate than conventional surgery [84].

Under anti-tuberculosis treatment, the course is usually favorable. Fever usually disappears within 2 weeks, but may persist for up to 2 months [12,67]. The complete resorption LP usually takes 6 to 12 weeks, but may take longer. This depends on the initial abundance of pleurisy. However, a paradoxical worsening of pleural effusion may in some cases after initiation of anti-tuberculosis treatment. Hiroaka et al have suggested that such paradoxical responses may be due to Isoniazid-induced lupus pleurisy [7, 22, 67, 85].

Two of our patients were lost to follow-up, and another patient was referred to his family. after diagnostic confirmation. Most patients

(n=46; 86%) showed regression of general signs within 15 days of starting treatment. After two months of anti-tuberculosis treatment, radiological improvement with a reduction in pleural opacity was noted in 31 patients (62% of cases), and complete radiological clearance in 9 patients (18% of cases). Cure was declared after 6 months of well-managed anti-tuberculosis treatment, with clinical and radiological improvement in 47 patients.

Despite well-administered anti-tuberculosis treatment, the incidence of pleural sequelae remains high, estimated in the literature at between 36% and 68% at the end of anti-tuberculosis treatment [82]. Significant sequelae have been defined by Han et al as residual pleural opacities whose width reaches or exceeds 10 mm at the end of treatment [81].

In this case, they may be responsible for functional respiratory repercussions in the form of a restrictive ventilatory disorder, the extent of which depends on the width of the residual pleural opacity [86].

Factors associated with the appearance of pleural thickening greater than 10 mm described in the literature were :

- Low glucose levels in the LP. Hypoglycopleuria could reflect elevated intrapleural bacterial activity, leading to increased pleural inflammation responsible for pleural sequelae [82].
- Low pleural Ph [87].
- A high concentration of lysozyme, TNF alpha and LDH in the LP [82,87].
- The presence of parenchymal lesions: In a Brazilian study, the presence of a parenchymal anomaly tripled the risk of developing significant residual pleural opacity at the end of anti-tuberculosis treatment [88].
- Smoking: this result described by Balkissou et al [82].

In our study, minimal sequelae were observed in 16 of our patients (32%), in the form of regular pleural thickening, occurring at an average delay of 6 months, and residual pleural effusion.

No statistically significant association was observed with the following parameters:

Smoking, the presence of parenchymal lesions on the initial radiograph, sexage over or under 60 years, time to consultation with respective p values of 0.6; 0.2; 0.9; 0.4; 0.7 and 0.8.

CONCLUSIONS

Extra-pulmonary tuberculosis attracted renewed interest in recent years due to its increasing frequency. Pleural tuberculosis is one of the most frequent forms of extra-pulmonary tuberculosis, and a common cause of pleural effusion, especially in countries with a high prevalence of tuberculosis. However, this form of tuberculosis has received little attention in the literature. In this context, we conducted a retrospective descriptive study over a 4-year period from January 2015 to December 2019, with the aim of describing the epidemiological, clinical and evolutionary profile of fifty cases of pleural tuberculosis managed in the Pneumology Department of Mohamed Taher Maamouri Hospital, Nabeul, as well as their therapeutic modalities.

Pleural TB affects young adults. The average age in our population was 40.4 years, and more than half our patients were between 20 and 50 years of age. No patient was HIV-positive, 7 patients were hypertensive, 3 patients were diabetic and 3 others had chronic renal failure at the hemodialysis stage.

Pleural TB is usually revealed by insidious respiratory and general symptoms. Respiratory symptoms were reported by all our patients, dominated by chest pain (80% of cases) and dyspnoea (32% of cases). General signs were present in 88% of cases. On chest X-ray, pleurisy was right-sided in 58% of cases, with parenchymal involvement in 5 patients.

Thoracic ultrasonography revealed partitions in favour of encystment in 9 cases. This examination is not systematic in cases of suspected pleural TB, but is recommended by the BTS in cases of small effusion or after failure of blind pleural puncture. Thoracic ultrasonography can also be used to guide pleural biopsy sites by showing localized pleural thickening or pleural nodules. This increases the cost-effectiveness of pleural sampling and reduces the risk of complications. This harmless, easy-to-perform test, which can be performed in the patient's own bed, should be considered before any pleural sampling. Young respirologists in training should encouraged to learn how to perform it.

Chest CT scans in 11 patients revealed associated parenchymal abnormalities such as subpleural micronodules and pleural thickening, undetected on chest X-ray in 2 patients.

A thoracic CT scan is not systematically performed in cases of suspected pleural TB . It is reserved for cases of diagnostic doubt or suspected complications, such as pleural empyema, since it enables better visualization of pleural and parenchymal abnormalities than standard radiography. It is also recommended as part of the preoperative work-up in cases where surgical sampling of the pleura is envisaged.

All patients underwent exploratory pleural puncture, except one, due to the fact that the multi-partitioned nature of his pleural effusion.

Pleural fluid was exudative, with a mean protid level of 53.45 g/L and lymphocytic predominance (lymphocyte/white cell count in pleural fluid > 50%) in all cases. Only one patient had a positive direct examination for BAARs in pleural fluid.

Blind pleural biopsy with the ABRAMS needle was performed in 47 patients (once in 44 patients, twice in 2 patients and three times in 1 patient), establishing the diagnosis in 46 cases. Surgical biopsy per thoracoscopy was performed immediately in 2 patients with compartmentalized pleurisy and after failure of a non-contributory blind biopsy in one patient.

In our study, a blind pleural biopsy was performed 51 times, enabling the diagnosis to be established in 46 cases, i.e. 90.1% cost-effectiveness. Complications of this procedure were noted in 6 patients: iatrogenic pneumothorax in 2 patients, which resolved with conservative measures, and vagal malaise in 4 patients.

Blind pleural biopsy is still widely used in developing countries, due to its low cost and accessibility, as well as its few and rare complications, dominated by iatrogenic pneumothorax, which rarely requires pleural evacuation and generally resolves spontaneously with conservative measures combining bed rest and high-concentration oxygen therapy.

Surgical pleural biopsy via thoracoscopy is the technique of choice for pleural sampling in developed countries. Its sensitivity is of the order of 100%, but at the cost of more complications and longer hospital stays. In our context, the use of this technique is limited by its cost and its unavailability in many hospitals. It is indicated in cases where bacteriological samples are negative, and if blind BP is non-contributory, or if it is not feasible due a linked to the patient's condition (haemostasis disorder , poor patient cooperation), or due to the compartmentalized nature of the effusion, preventing blind biopsies. Classically, two BPs are often recommended before indicating surgical thoracoscopy.

In recent years, other molecular biology or immuno-biochemical methods have been developed to confirm the tuberculous nature of pleural effusions, particularly in industrialized countries. However, their use is limited in developing countries, as is the case in our context, due to their high cost and unavailability.

All patients received the anti-tuberculosis treatment prescribed by national anti-tuberculosis program. The standard regimen of isoniazid-rifampicin-ethambutol and pyrazinamide for two months, followed by isoniazid and rifampicin for four months, was used in 44 patients. Pleural fluid evacuation was necessary in 35 patients: by evacuation puncture in 34 cases and by surgical drainage in one case. Pleural softening physiotherapy was followed in 94% of cases.

Two of our patients were lost to follow-up, while another was referred back to his home department diagnostic confirmation. Cure was declared for the other 47 patients at the end of treatment, with clinical and radiological improvement. Sixteen patients (32%) retained radiological sequelae such as pleural thickening or residual pleural effusion. There was no statistically significant association between the appearance of these sequelae and the patient's smoking status, gender, age under or over 60, or the presence of associated parenchymal lesions on the first chest X-ray. The functional impact of these sequelae has not been studied.

Treatment of pleural TB is based on a combination of several anti-tuberculosis drugs, often lasting up to 6 months. Some authors have suggested systematic corticosteroid therapy in the initial phase, in cases of intense general signs. Pleural evacuation is only indicated in cases of poor clinical tolerance of pleural effusion. Early pleural physiotherapy is essential reduce the incidence of pleural sequelae.

In view of these results, we can draw the following conclusions:

- Pleural TB should be suspected in the presence of any lymphocytic pleural effusion in young subjects, particularly in developing countries.

- Blind pleural biopsy is a cost-effective technique for diagnosing pleural TB. It is widely used in developing countries, due to its cost and accessibility. Complications are rare and mild. However, its use is becoming limited in our country due to the non-availability of biopsy forceps, which are no longer on the market. Local production of this needle should therefore be considered by the health authorities, particularly as it is a simple device to manufacture.
- Thoracic ultrasound prior to pleural sampling should be encouraged, to increase the cost-effectiveness of sampling and reduce the incidence of complications. Young respirologists in training should be encouraged to learn how to perform this technique.
- The incidence of pleural sequelae such pleural thickening more than 10mm remains high, estimated at 32% in our study. Smoking status, sex, age under or over 60 and the presence of initial parenchymal lesions did not influence the appearance of these sequelae.

However, the effect of continuing physiotherapy after hospital discharge has not been studied, and needs to be the subject of larger studies. In addition, the respiratory functional impact of these sequelae needs to be studied, so that respiratory rehabilitation programs can be proposed in good time.

REFERENCES

1. World Health Organization. Global tuberculosis report 2021 [Online]. 2021 [cited May 25, 2022]. Available from: https://www.who.int/publications/i/item/9789240037021

2. Ketata W, Rekik WK, Ayadi H, Kammoun S. Les tuberculoses extrapulmonaires. Rev Pneumol Clin. Apr 2015;71(2-3):83-92.

3. World Health Organization. New case notifications: data by country [Online]. 2020 [cited June 17, 2022]. Available from: https://worldhealthorg.shinyapps.io/tb_profiles

4. Direction des Soins de Santé de Base. Le guide national de prise en charge de la tuberculose en tunisie-2018 [Online]. 2018 [cited May 25, 2022]. Available from: http://www.santetunisie.rns.tn/fr/toutes-les-actualites/807-dssb-le-guide- national-de-prise-en-charge-de-la-tuberculose-%C3%A9dition-2018

5. Zorai R. Clinical and radiological manifestations of extra pulmonary tuberculosis [Thesis]. Medicine: Tunis; 2018. 78p.

6. Antonangelo L, Faria C, Sales R. Tuberculous pleural effusion: diagnosis and management. Expert Rev Respir Med. 2019 Aug;13(8):747-59.

7. Vorster MJ, Allwood BW, Diacon AH, Koegelenberg CF. Tuberculous pleural effusions: advances and controversies. J Thorac Dis. Jun 2015;7(6):981-91.

8. Greillier L, Peloni JM, Fraticelli A, Astoul P. Methods for investigating the pleura. EMC-Pneumology. 2005;2(3):127-146

9. Zhai K, Lu Y, Shi HZ. Tuberculous pleural effusion. J Thorac Dis. Mar 2016;8(7):486-94

10. Bemba EP, Moukassa D, Ouedraogo AR, Okemba Okombi FH, Bopaka RG, Koumeka PP, et al. Performance of GeneXpert MTB/RIF in the diagnosis of pleural tuberculosis in Brazzaville: preliminary study. Health Sci Dis. August 2017;18(3):21-7.

11. Munavvar M, Khan MA, Edwards J, Waqaruddin Z, Mills J. The autoclavable semirigid thoracoscope: the way forward in pleural disease? Eur Respir J. 2007 Mar;29(3):571-4.

12. Udwadia ZF, Sen T. Pleural tuberculosis: an update. Curr Opin Pulm Med. 2010 Jul;16(4):399-406.

13. Ouédraogo M, Ki C, Ouédraogo SM, Zoubga AZ, Badoum G, Zigani A, et al. Epidemio-

clinical aspects of serofibrinous pleurisy at the Yalgado Ouedraogo National Hospital. Med Afr Noire. Mar 2000;(47):386-89.

14. Koffi N, Aka Danguy E, Kouassi B, Ngom A, Blehou DJ. Les étiologies des pleurésies en milieu africain: l'expérience du service de pneumologie de Cocody. Rev Pneumol Clin. Mar 1997;53(4):193-6.

15. Ossalé Abacka KB, Koné A, Akoli Ekoya O, Bopaka RG, Lankoandé Siri H, Horo K, et al. Extrapulmonary versus pulmonary tuberculosis: epidemiological, diagnostic and evolutionary aspects. Rev Pneumol Clin. Apr 2018;(74):452-57.

16. Light RW. Tuberculous pleural effusion [Online]. 2015 [cited May 25, 2022]. Available About: www.msdmanuals.com/fr/professional/troubles- https://pulmonary/disorders-m%C3%A9diastinal-and-pleural/fibrosis-and-pleural-calcifications.

17. Ben Ghars K. Epidemiological, clinical and evolutionary aspects of extra-pulmonary tuberculosis: about 95 cases [Thesis]. Medicine: Tunis; 2007. 116p.

18. Ajmi T, Tarmiz H, Bougmiza I, Gataa R, Knani H, Mtiraoui A. Epidemiological profile of tuberculosis in the Sousse health region from 1995 to 2005. Revue Tunisienne d'Infectiologie. Jan 2010;4:18-22.

19. Ouardi O, Sajiai H, Serhane H, Ait Batahar S, Amro L. Tuberculous pleurisy. J Func Vent Pulm. May 2016;20(7):15-18.

20. Pefura Yone EW, Kuaban C, Simo L. Tuberculous pleurisy in Yaoundé, Cameroon: influence of HIV infection. Rev Mal Respir. Nov 2011;28(9):1138- 45.

21. Aazri L. Prise en charge de la tuberculose extra-pulmonaire: expérience du service de pneumologie de l'hôpital militaire avicenne de Marrakech [Thesis]. Medicine: Marrakech; 2018. 144p.

22. Shaw JA, Irusen EM, Diacon AH, Koegelenberg CF. Pleural tuberculosis: a concise clinical review. Clin Respir J. May 2018;12(5):1779-86.

23. Lian CK, Lim KH, Wong CM. Tuberculous pleurisy as a manifestation of primary reactivation in an area of high tuberculosis prevalence. Int J Tuberc Lung Dis. Sep 1999;3(9):816-22.

24. Randriatsarafara FM, Vololonarivelo BE, Rabemananjara NN, Randrianasolo JB, Rakotomanga JD, Randrianarimanana VD. Factors associated with tuberculosis in children at the mother-child university hospital of Tsaralalàna, antananarivo: a case-control study. Pan Afr Med J. Oct 2014;19:224.

25. Poinsignon Y, Marjanovic Z, Bordon P , Georges C, Farge D. Re-emergence of tuberculosis and socioeconomic precariousness. Rev Med Interne. Sep 1998;19(9):649- 57.

26. Emmanuelli X, Grosset J. Tuberculose and poverty. Rev Mal Respir. Mar 2008;20(2):169-71.

27. Lacut JY, Dupon M, Paty MC. Extra-pulmonary tuberculosis: review and possibilities for reducing therapeutic response times. Med Mal Infect. Mar 1995;25(3):304-20.

28. Tsevi MY, Lawson Ananissoh LM, Sabi K, Kadou Kaza BN. Tuberculosis in chronic hemodialysis patients in Togo: about 10 observations. Nephrol Ther. Feb 2017;13(1):14-7.

29. Chakroun M, Razik F, Karkouri M, Fall Malick Z, Benothman H, George Hermez J. The HIV epidemic in the greater Maghreb: magnitude, trend and management. Tunis Med. 2018;96(10):599-605.

30. El Amrani M, Asserraji M, Bahadi A, El Kabbaj D, Benyahia M. Tuberculosis in hemodialysis. Med Sante Trop. 2016 Aug;26(3):262-6.

31. Cherif J, Mjid M, Ladhar A, Toujani S, Mokadem S, Louzir B, et al. Diagnostic delay in pulmonary and pleural tuberculosis. Rev Pneumol Clin. Aug 2014;70(4):189-94.

32. Odusanya OO, Babafemi JO. Patterns of delays amongst pulmonary tuberculosis patients in Lagos, Nigeria. BMC Public Health. 2004 May;4:18.

33. Pronyk RM , Makhubele MB, Hargreaves JR, Tollman SM, Hausler HP. Assessing health seeking behaviour among tuberculosis patients in rural South Africa. Int J Tuberc Lung Dis. 2001 Jul;5(7):619-27.

34. Leung EC, Leung CC, Tam CM. Delayed presentation and treatment of newly diagnosed pulmonary tuberculosis patients in Hong Kong. Hong Kong Med J. 2007 Jun;13(3):221-7.

35. Lo Cascio CM, Kaul V, Dhooria S, Agrawal A, Chaddha U. Diagnosis of tuberculous pleural effusions: a review. Respir Med. 2021 Nov;188:106607.

36. Shaw JA, Diacon AH, Koegelenberg CN. Tuberculous pleural effusion. Respirology. 2019 Oct;24(10):962-71.

37. Du Rand I, Maskell N. Introduction and methods: british thoracic society pleural disease guideline 2010. Thorax. 2010 Aug;65 Suppl 2:1-3.

38. Ko JM, Park HJ, Kim CH. Pulmonary changes in pleural tuberculosis. Chest. Jan 2014;146(6):1604-11.

39. Kim HJ, Lee HJ, Kwon SY, Yoon HI, Chung HS, Lee CT, et al. The prevalence of pulmonary parenchymal tuberculosis in patients with tuberculous pleuritis. Chest. 2006 May;129(5):1253-8.

40. Mollo B, Jouveshomme S, Philippart F, Pilmis B. Biomarkers for the diagnosis of tuberculous pleurisy. Ann Biol Clin. Feb 2017;75(1):19-27.

41. Epstein DM, Kline LR, Albelda SM, Miller WT. Tuberculous pleural effusions. Chest. 1987 Jan;91(1):106-9.

42. Heyderman RS, Makunike R, Muza T, Odwee M, Kadzirange G, Manyemba J, et al. Pleural tuberculosis in Harare, Zimbabwe: the relationship between human immunodeficiency virus, CD4 lymphocyte count, granuloma formation and disseminateddisease. Trop Med Int Health. 1998 Jan;3(1):14-20.

43. Scheicher ME, Terra Filho J, Vianna EO. Sputum induction: review of literature and proposal for a protocol. Sao Paulo Med J. 2003 Sep;121(5):213-9.

44. Conde MB, Loivos AC, Rezende VM, Soares SL, Mello FC, Reingold AL, et al. Yield of sputum induction in the diagnosis of pleural tuberculosis. Am J Respir Crit Care Med. 2003 Mar;167(5):723-5.

45. Groupe de Travail du Conseil Supérieur d'Hygiène Publique, France. Prevention of tuberculosis transmission in health care facilities. Med Mal Infect. Aug 2004;34(8):404-10.

46. Berger HW, Mejia E. Tuberculous pleurisy. Chest. 1973 Jan;63(1):88-92.

47. Groote Bidlingmaier FV, Koegelenberg CF, Bolliger CT, Khi Chung P, Rautenbach C, Wasserman E, et al. The yield of different pleural fluid volumes for mycobacterium tuberculosis culture. Thorax. 2013 Mar;68(3):290-1.

48. Bernaudin JF, scherpereel A, Rekik WK, Hussenet C. Pleural fluid analysis: first-line orientation. Rev Malad Respir Actual. Jan 2013;(5):168-71.

49. Babalik A, Kiziltas S, Oruc K, Cetintas G, Altunbey S, Haluk C, et al. The profile of pleural tuberculosis patients in Turkey. Med Sci. 2013 May;2(1):374-85.

50. Sharma SK, Mohan A. Extrapulmonary tuberculosis. Indian J Med Res. 2004 Oct;120(4):316-53.

51. Berger HW, Mejra E. Tuberculous pleurisy. Chest. 1973 Jan;63(1):88-92.

52. Maartens G, Bateman ED. Tuberculous pleural effusions increased yield with besides inoculation of pleural fluid and poor diagnostic value of adenosine deaminase. Thorax. 1991 Feb;46(2):96-9.

53. Toloba Y, Diallo S, Sissoko BF, Kamaté B, Ouattara K, Somaré D, et al. Pleural biopsy puncture in the etiologic diagnosis of pleurisy. Rev Mal Respir. Sep 2011;28(7):881-4.

54. Kirsch CM, Jensen WA, Kagawa FT, Wehner JH, Kroe DM, Azzi RL. The optimal number of pleural biopsy specimens for a diagnosis of tuberculous pleurisy. Chest. 1997 Sep;112(3):702-6.

55. Baslam S. The contribution of thoracoscopy in the diagnosis of pleurisy [Thesis]. Medicine: Rabat; 2016. 162p.

56. Ngom A, Koffi N, Aka Danguy E, Kouakou KJ, Sanou R, Diallo M, et al. Apport de la biopsie pleurale au diagnostic des pleurésies tuberculeuses et étude prospective de 89 cas au CHU d'Abidjan. Med Afr Noire. Nov 1997;44(2):81-3.

57. Duysinx B, Heinen V, Corhay JL, Vaillant F, Gomez A, Louis R. La thoracoscopie médicale en pratique pneumologique : expérience du CHU de liége. Rev Mal Respir. Jun 2019;36(6):688-96.

58. Mehta PK, Raj A, Singh N, Khuller GK. Diagnosis of extrapulmonary tuberculosis by

PCR. FEMS Immunol Med Microbiol. 2012 Oct;66(1):20-36.

59. Pai M, Flores LL, Hubbard A, Riley LW, Colford JM. Nucleic acid amplification tests in the diagnosis of tuberculous pleuritis: a systematic review and meta-analysis. BMC Infect Dis. 2004 Feb;4:6.

60. World Health Organization. WHO Unified Guidelines on Tuberculosis. Module 2: screening. Routine screening for tuberculosis [Online]. 2022 [cited 2022 May 25]; [72 pages]. Available from: https://apps.who.int/iris/bitstream/handle/10665/353406/9789240047969-fre.pdf

61. Le Paluda P, Herrman JL, Bergota E. Interferon gamma assays (IGRA). Rev Mal Respir. Oct 2018;35(8):862-5.

62. Smach MA, Garouch A, Charfeddine B, Abdelaziz AB, Dridi H, Krayem B, et al. Diagnostic value of pleural and serum adenosine deaminase activity in tuberculous pleurisy. Ann Biol Clin. May 2006;64(3):265-70.

63. Junyun H, Zhang R, Yongchun S, Chun W, Zeng N, Jiangyue Q, et al. Diagnostic accuracy of interleukin-22 and adenosine deaminase for tuberculous pleural effusions. Curr Res Transl Med. 2018 Nov;66(4):103-6.

64. Gopi A, Madhavan SM, Sharma SK, Sahn SA. Diagnosis and treatment of tuberculous pleural effusion in 2006. Chest. 2007 Mar;131(3):880-9

65. Garcia Pachon E, Soler M, Padilla Navas I, Romero V, Shum C. C-reactive protein in lymphocytic pleural effusions: a diagnostic aid in tuberculous pleuritis. Respiration. 2005 Sep;72(5):486-9.

66. Xirouchaki N, Tzanakis N, Bouros D, Kyriakou D, Karkavitsas N, Alexandrakis M, et al. Diagnostic value of interleukin-1alpha, interleukin-6, and tumor necrosis factor in pleural effusions. Chest. 2002 Mar;121(3):815-20.

67. Doosoo J. Tuberculous pleurisy: an update. Tuberc Respir Dis. 2014 Apr;76(4):153-9.

68. World Health Organization. Guidelines for the treatment and management of drug-susceptible tuberculosis [Online]. 2017 [cited 2022 May 25]; [80 pages]. Available from: https://apps.who.int/iris/bitstream/handle/10665/258933/9789242550009-fre.pdf

69. Canete C, Galarza M , Granados U, Farrero E, Estopa R, Manrèse F. Tuberculous pleural effusion: experiencewith six months of treatment with isoniazid and rifampicin. Thorax. 1994 Nov;49(11):1160-1.

70. Dutt AK, Moers D, Stead WW. Tuberculous pleural effusion: 6-month therapy with isoniazid and rifampin. Am Rev Respir Dis. 1992 Jun;145(6):1429-32.

71. Wyser C, Walzl G, Smédema JP, Swart F, Schalkwyk EV, Van De Wal BW. Corticosteroids in the treatment of tuberculous pleurisy: a double-blind, placebo controlled, randomized study. Chest. 1996 Aug;110(2):333-8.

72. Galarza I, Cañete C, Granados A, Estopà R, Manresa F. Randomized trial of corticosteroids in the treatment of tuberculous pleurisy. Thorax. Dec 1995;50(12):1305-7.

73. Lee CH, Wang WJ, Lan RS, Tsai YH, Chiang YC. Corticosteroids in the treatment of tuberculous pleurisy. A double-blind, placebo-controlled, randomized study. Chest. 1988 Dec;94(6):1256-9.

74. Engel ME, Matchaba PT, Volmink J. Corticosteroids for tuberculous pleurisy. Cochrane Database Syst Rev. 2007 Oct;(4):CD001876.

75. Bhuniya S, Arunabha DC, Choudhury S, Saha I, Roy TS, Saha M. Role of therapeutic thoracentesis in tuberculous pleural effusion. Ann Thorac Med. 2012 Oct;7(4):215- 9.

76. Cases Viedma E, Lorenzo Dus MJ, Gonzalez Molina A, Sanchis Aldas JL. A study of loculated tuberculous pleural effusions treated with intrapleural urokinase. Respir Med. 2006 Nov;100(11):2037-42.

77. Kwak SM, Park CS, Cho JH, Ryu JS, Kim SK, Chang J, et al. The effects of urokinase instillation therapy via percutaneous transthoracic catheter in loculated tuberculous pleural effusion: a randomized prospective study. Yonsei Med J. 2004 Oct;45(5):822-8.

78. Souhi H, El Ouazzani H, Janah H, Rhorfi I, Abid A. Tuberculous pyo-pneumothorax: at About 18 cases. Pan Afr Med J. May 2016;24:26.

79. Horo K, Gom A, Ahui B, Brougode C, Anon JC, Diaw A, et al. Non-tuberculous pleural infections versus tuberculous pleural infections. Rev Mal Respir. 2012 Mar;29(3):404-11.

80. Charafi Z. Pyothorax surgery [Thesis]. Medicine: Marrakech; 2017. 138p.

81. Han DH, Song JW, Chung HS, Lee JH. Resolution of residual pleural diseaseaccording to time course in tuberculous pleurisy during and after the termination of antituberculosis medication. Chest. 2005 Nov;128(5):3240-5.

82. Balkissou AD, Perfura Yone EW, Netong Gamgne M, Endale Mangamba LM, Onana Ngono I, Poka Mayab V et al. Residual pleural opacity at the end of treatment for pleural tuberculosis in Yaoundé. Rev Pneumol Clin. Apr 2016;72(2):115-21.

83. Kilani T, Boudaya MS, Zribi H, Ouerghi S, Marghli A, Mestiri T, et al. Surgery in thoracic tuberculosis. Rev Pneumol Clin. Apr 2015;71(2-3):140-58.

84. Bernard A, Migueres M, Jaillard S, Gibelin A. Decortication: techniques, indications, results. Rev Malad Respir Actual. Jan 2013;(5):127-30.

85. Hiraoka K, Nagata N, Kawajiri T, Suzuki K, Kurokawa S, Kido M, et al. Paradoxical pleural response to antituberculous chemotherapy and isoniazid-induced lupus. Review and report of two cases. Respiration. 1998 Sep;65(2):152-5.

86. Candela A, Andujar J, Hernández L, Martín C, Barroso E, Arriero JM. Functional sequelae of tuberculous pleurisy in patients correctly treated. Chest. 2003 Jun;123(6):1996-2000.

87. Wong PC. Management of tuberculous pleurisy: can we do better? Respirology. Feb 2005;10(2)144-8.

88. Seiscento M, Vargas FS, Bombarda S, Sales RK, Terra RM, Uezumi K, et al. Pulmonary involvement in pleural tuberculosis: how often does it mean disease activity? Respir Med. 2011 Jul;105(7):1079-83.

APPENDICES

Pleural tuberculosis data sheet

I. Identity :

-Full name:........

-Age :....

-Gender: male..... Female......

-Residence : * resident in Tunisia .... *not resident in Tunisia......

*resident at cap bon.... (Delegation : ………………)

*outside cape bon.....

-Living environment : rural ..... urban ......

-profession : blue-collar .... liberal profession .... Civil servant ...... Retired .....

no profession ..... unspecified ......

-Schooling : not in school ..... primary level .... secondary level.....

higher education ...... not specified .....

-Socio-economic level : good ..... average .... Poor ..... unspecified .....

-History incarceration: yes ..... No .....

II. Background:

1. Employees

-BCG vaccination: yes .... No .... Not specified ....

-History of tuberculosis: ....

* Pulmonary tuberculosis .....

* Extra pulmonary .....

If yes, location:...........

*No recent tuberculosis contagion (less than 2 years) ......

-Medication : immunosuppressant ..... corticosteroid therapy ......

Cancer chemotherapy ......

-Other associated pathologies: Diabetes : ......

Chronic renal failure: .....

Associated neoplasia: .....

Hepatitis B/C: .... Other:........

2. Toxic habits :

-Tobacco: yes .... No .... Not specified .....

-Type of tobacco: cigarette ......

chicha personal use ..... Shisha for public use .....

-Alcohol: yes ..... No ..... Not specified .....

-drug addiction ....

Other:........

3. Family :

*Pulmonary tuberculosis .... *Extrapulmonary tuberculosis ...

*Others:.....

III. Diagnosis of pleural tuberculosis

1) Reason for consultation:.....

2) Consultation deadline:......

3) clinical signs :

No signs: ...... Accidental discovery during a check-up

4. Biological tests :

CBC: Hb:..... GB : .... Lym : ..... Plq : ....

VS : ... CRP: ... Urea : .... Creat : ....

Transaminases: ASAT: ... ALAT: ... Electrolyte disorders:.......

5. Tuberculin TST :

-positive ☐ induration diameter ....

-negative ☐

-not done ☐

-result not specified ☐

6. Radiological examination :

Rx thorax:		Radiological aspects:	
location pleural effusion :			
-Right	☐	-freepleuresis	☐
-Left	☐	-cloisonnepleuresis	☐
-Bilateral	☐	-hydro PNO	☐
Abundance of pleural effusion :		-associated parenchymal	
-low CDS blunting		tuberculosis lesions	☐
-average <1 /3 CP			
large> 1/3 CP			

Trans-thoracic ultrasound		Sonographic aspects :	
-Made	☐	-freepleuresis	☐
-Not made	☐	-cloisonnepleuresis	☐
		-pleural thickening	☐

Chest CT	Aspects of CT :	
-Done: ...	-liquid seal	☐
-Not done: ...	-mixed joint	☐
	-free branching	☐
	-partitioned joint	☐
	- Associated mediastinal ADP	☐
	Calcified yes no	
	- associated parenchymal TBC lesion	☐

5. Means of diagnostic confirmation :

5-1 pleural puncture

* Macroscopic appearance:...

* Biochemistry: exudate:...transudate :....

* Cytology: WBC:... PNN :.... Lc:..

*ADA: ...

Direct examination:.... Culture:.....

5-2 Pleural biopsy: * Caseous necrosis:....

* Tuberculoid granuloma: .... * Necrosis and granuloma:.....

6. Diagnostic delay:...

Year of diagnosis ...... Month of diagnosis......

IV. Treatment of pleural tuberculosis :

1. drug therapy :

1-1 Pre-therapy assessment :

Ophthalmic examination:	Liver function tests :	Uric acid :	HIV serology :
Fact .....non fact .... Normal:yes .....non..... Type fault.....	Fact .....non fact .... Normal:yes .....non..... Type fault.....	Fact .....non fact .... Normal:yes .....non..... Type fault.....	Made ... not made .... Positive.... Negative ....

1-2 anti-bacillary treatment

Duration of treatment: 2-month	
treatment: 1)combined(HRZE) ☐ 2) dissociated ☐ Treatment dose: 1)2cp 2)3cp 3)4cp 4)5cp 5)dissociated treatment	Compliance: good ☐ Poor Unspecified ☐ Reasons for non-compliance : ☐ -poor relationship with the health worker: -the patient no longer feels ill: ☐ ☐ -stigmatization (fear or refusal of being seen as a tuberculosis): ☐ -alcoholism or drug addiction : - other negligence : ☐

Monitoring of side effects :		Types of side effects :
-audiogram :	☐	-hepatic cytolysis: 5-10N :
liver check-up :	☐	>10N :
renal check-up :	☐	-hepatic cholestasis :
-uric acid :	☐	-Moderate skin rash (pruritus):
-ophthalmologic examination :	☐	-nausea, vomiting:
-Acetylation :	☐	-arthralgias :
		-peripheral neuropathies :
1) slow	☐	-red-orange coloring of tears, urine :
2) fast	☐	-auditory toxicity :
3) not done	☐	-vestibular toxicity :
4) unspecified	☐	

Presence of side effects: yes on

Time onset of side effects:......

-nephrotoxicity :

-optical neuritis :

-other: ......

1-3 symptomatic treatment :

High-protein nutrition: ....

-Correction of electrolytic disorders: ....

-oxygen therapy: ....

-mechanical ventilation: ....

2. Non-medicinal treatment :

-pleural physiotherapy ....

-evacuating punctures ....

-pleural decortications .....

3. associated measures : Declaration:.....

Inquiry in entourage :.....

Work stoppage: ....

Financial assistance:.......

V. Evolution :

- Healing
- Weight gain
- Improved general condition (improvement in asthenia and anorexia)
- Treatment failure: yes / no

Rx thorax control: 1month ....2 months.... 3months....4months .... 5months..... 6months ....

BK control: 1month ....2months.... 3months....4months .... 5months..... 6months ....

End-of-treatment chest x-ray :

*normal ....

*Sequelle: ...

*presence pleural effusion of lesser or equal abundance: ...

*pleural thickening: ....

*other

PLEURAL TUBERCULOSIS: EPIDEMIOLOGICAL, CLINICAL AND EVOLUTIONARY ASPECTS

Summary

Introduction:

Pleural tuberculosis is one of the most common forms of extrapulmonary tuberculosis. Its incidence has been steadily increasing in recent years. However, this form of tuberculosis is little studied in the literature.

The purpose of our study was to study the epidemiological, clinical and evolutionary profile of pleural tuberculosis in the Cap Bon region and its treatment modalities.

Method:

We conducted a retrospective descriptive study of 50 records of patients with pleural tuberculosis who were diagnosed and monitored in the pneumology department of the Mohamed Taher Maamouri Hospital over a 4year period from January 2015 to Decemb er 2019.

Results:

The average age of our population was 40.4 years. Signs of appeal were dominated by respiratory symptoms (chest pain in 80% of cases; cough in 68% of cases). Chest X- ray objectified pleural opacity in all cases; on the right side in 58% of cases. The diagnosis of pleural tuberculosis was made by Acid fast bacili identification on direct examination of pleural fluid for a single patient.

For the remaining 49 cases, the diagnosis was confirmed by a pleural biopsy: Needle blind in 46 cases and surgical thoracoscopy in 3 cases.

Tuberculosis treatment according to the guidelines of the National Tuberculosis Control Program was initiated in all cases, in combination with pleural relaxation.

physiotherapy in 47 cases and pleural evacuation in 35 patients.

Three patients were lost to sight. Healing was achieved in all other cases. Radiological sequelae were noted in 16 patients.

Conclusion:

Pleural tuberculosis should be considered before any lymphocytic effusion of the young subject especially in developing countries.

His clinic is not very specific.

The diagnosis is often histological in view of the paucibacillary nature of pleural effusion Blind pleural biopsy is a cost-effective method of diagnosing with rare and mild comlications. The evolution is usually favorable under well-conducted treatment Keywords:

Pleural tuberculosis, Epidemiology, Therapy, Evolution.

PLEURAL TUBERCULOSIS: EPIDEMIOLOGICAL, CLINICAL AND EVOLUTIONARY ASPECTS

Summary

Introduction :

Pleural tuberculosis is one of the most common extra-pulmonary tuberculoses. Its incidence has been rising steadily in recent years. However, this form of tuberculosis has received little attention in the literature. The aim of our study was to investigate the epidemiological, clinical and evolutionary profile of pleural tuberculosis in the Cap Bon region, as well as its therapeutic modalities.

Methods :

We conducted a descriptive retrospective study of 50 records of patients with pleural tuberculosis who were diagnosed and followed at the Pneumology Department of the Mohamed Taher Maamouri Nabeul University Hospital Center over a 4-year period from January 2015 until December 2019.

Results :

The average age of our population was 40.4 years. The presenting signs were dominated by respiratory symptoms (chest pain in 80% of cases; cough in 68%). Chest radiography revealed a pleural opacity in all cases; right in 58%. The diagnosis of pleural tuberculosis was established by the presence of acid-fast bacilli on direct examination of the LP in only one patient. For the remaining 49 cases, the diagnosis was confirmed by pleural biopsy: blind needle biopsy in 46 cases and surgical thoracoscopy in 3 cases. Anti-tuberculosis treatment in accordance with the guidelines of the national anti-tuberculosis program was instituted in all cases, combined with pleural relaxation physiotherapy in 47 cases and pleural evacuation in 35 patients. Two of our patients were lost to follow-up. Another patient was referred back to his original department after diagnostic confirmation. Recovery was achieved in all other cases. Radiological sequelae were noted in 16 patients.

Conclusion:

Pleural tuberculosis should be suspected in young people with lymphocytic effusions, particularly in developing countries. Its clinical features are not very specific. Diagnosis is often histological, given the paucibacillary nature of the pleural effusion. Blind pleural biopsy is a cost-effective technique for establishing the diagnosis, with rare and mild complications. The course is usually favorable under well-managed treatment.

Keywords: Pleural tuberculosis, Epidemiology, Treatment, Evolution

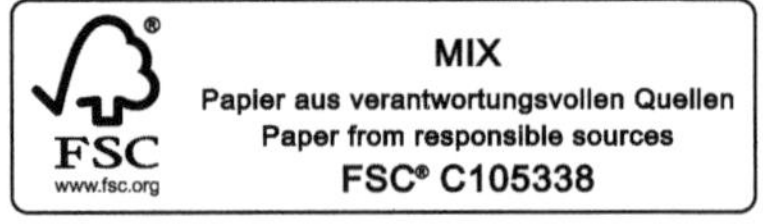

Printed by Books on Demand GmbH, Norderstedt / Germany